# GOLD

## *CATALYST OF RADIANT HEALTH*

By

VICTOR SAGALOVSKY

Copyright © 2005 – 2018

## *Legal Notes*

Copyright © 2005-2018 Victor Sagalovsky

ALL RIGHTS RESERVED.

This Book contains materials protected under Copyright Law and Treaties. Any unauthorized reprint or use of this material is highly prohibited.

No part of this publication may be reproduced, distributed, or transmitted in any form or by any means, including photocopying, recording, or other electronic or mechanical methods, without the prior written permission of the publisher or Author, except in the case of brief quotations embodied in reviews and certain other non-commercial uses permitted by copyright law

First Publication, 2016

## DISCLAIMER

This book is written for information purposes only. Every effort was made to make this book as complete and accurate as possible. This book provides information only up to the publishing date. Therefore, this book should be used as a guide - not as the ultimate source.

The purpose of this book is to educate. The author and the publisher do not warrant that the information contained in this book is fully complete and shall not be responsible for any errors or omissions. The author and publisher shall have neither liability nor responsibility to any person or entity with respect to any loss or damage caused or alleged to be caused directly or indirectly by this book.

## *Table of Contents*

| | | |
|---|---|---|
| Preface | ------------------- | 1 |
| Introduction | ------------------- | 8 |
| What is Gold? | ------------------- | 10 |
| What Makes Gold Non-Metallic? | ------------------- | 12 |
| Gold + Silica = Aurosilica | ------------------- | 22 |
| Real Gold ORMUS vs. Fake | ------------------- | 25 |
| How We Make It | ------------------- | 27 |
| Historical Uses | ------------------- | 32 |
| Modern Uses | ------------------- | 38 |
| A Review of Benefits | ------------------- | 45 |
| The Harvard Study | ------------------- | 49 |
| Skin Rejuvenation | ------------------- | 52 |
| How to Use on Skin | ------------------- | 55 |
| Gold with Light Therapy | ------------------- | 57 |
| Brain Health | ------------------- | 60 |
| Gold as Aphrodisiac | ------------------- | 63 |
| Evidence of Gold's Therapeutic Use in Bible | | 65 |
| Conclusion + Bonus | ------------------- | 67 |
| Bonus 1: 'Tractatus Aureus' | ------------------- | 69 |
| Bonus 2: The Book of Revelation of Hermes | | 88 |
| Bibliography | ------------------- | 100 |

*Light is the instrument of the soul.*

*The art of your life is the art of light,*

*The language of light is the first language.*

*Deep down in your genes,*

*DNA emits coherent structured light,*

*a communication system between cells.*

*Alchemical Gold enhances that light.*

*It allows Mind to exist in this dimension.*

*21 grams of your body weight leaves*

*at the moment of death. What is it?*

# Preface

Gold, known to the ancients as the metal of the gods, is the symbol of love, fidelity and purity, the icon of all that is sacred and noble.

Gold, being a transition element, is quite synonymous with the times in which we live; a world in upheaval and transition. Humanity is on the brink of a rebirth into a higher level of consciousness, yearning for a new awareness that will save us from self-destruction in the eleventh hour.

In nature, gold is never found pure, so it must be refined just like us, just like everything; we strip away the inessentials until the essence is revealed.

Gold is the only known element that is impervious to moisture, oxygen or ordinary acids. And though virtually indestructible and immutable, it is a soft metal, easy to work with, shape, flatten or draw out. A very small amount can be made into a microscopic strand many miles long.

Because of its color, it is universally associated as related to the Sun, our cosmic source of life. Thus, gold is awarded the attributes of excellence, radiance, clarity, vitality, virtue, and light.

I first became interested in the therapeutic use of gold at the turn of the 20th century. I was living in a health-conscious community in Hawaii. I was suffering from mercury poisoning, kundalini awakening and other afflictions of an Indigo child in the modern world. I was in my 20's and voracious for knowledge and experience. As an immigrant kid from the Soviet Union growing up in Chicago, I seemed pretty normal to others, but I hid a rich inner world of spiritual seeking I didn't share within anyone until much later. By my early twenties I had reinvented myself as a barefoot yogi raw foodist living off the land in Kaua`i studying the wonders of life, pursuing the non material riches, bent on cosmic initiation and self realization. I devoured books on esoteric knowledge like an apex predator at the point of starvation. With my deep desire for wisdom I was fortunate to attract the teachers and elders whose lessons and teachings shaped my understanding. In time I had received the mystical experiences I had craved. And so in these formative years in the late 90's I came across writings about a sacred white powder made of gold that had magical properties. I cross correlated many texts referencing this "philosopher's stone". One story in particular was on the internet at the time and it was the story of David Radius Hudson and his rediscovery of ORMUS.

I began networking within the nascent online ORMUS community, a precocious cadre of lovable weirdos that spoke my language; the self-proclaimed alchemists, metaphysicians, and psychedelic voyagers rediscovering the secrets of the ancients. This group was not interested in academic pursuits, science was a only a tool to push beyond its limits in the pursuit of exotic matter.

I was attracted to ORMUS because I first had read that it could purify the karmic body and bring you closer to God, that it had an amplifying effect that can make spiritual progress faster, that it could stimulate mystical experience, either remembering past lives, bi-locating, awakening telekinesis, superpowers, you name it. Even if this was fantasy. I was all in.

To the ancients, evidence is without a doubt, these types of alchemical preparations, especially from gold, were regarded as nourishment for the spirit, conferring wisdom, aligning the astral, causal, and physical bodies, purifying the soul, increasing life force and extending the lifespan. If the ancient Sumerians, Hebrews, Egyptians and aliens were into it, certainly it was meant for me as well. Through mere luck or providence, I was able to receive a small sample of ORMUS from a legit source, an reclusive hobby alchemist tinkering for a decade in his lab on the quest for the philosopher's stone. He made it clear there would be no more after that first sample, he was making it for people with serious terminal illnesses, and even then he said not for much longer because he was going on a long trip, whatever that meant.

I ended up having quite the life changing and memorable experience ingesting that powder he gave me, and that's putting it mildly. Now I'm not going to go into what that was in this book because its doubtful anyone would believe me if I did. Let's just say that half gram of powder I can credit for being the catalyst for an abrupt and fateful shift in the events in my life. I can also give it credit for mobilizing the mercury I was poisoned with from a young age out of my brain. I learned to respect it like it was fire or a live wire.

After my profound healing experience with this substance I had never heard of before I naturally wanted to get more. Some of the names alchemical gold and altered spin state monatomic elements have been called by many names including ORMUS, ORME, monatomic gold, high-spin state elements, aurum potabile, manna, mfkzt, shem-manna, white powder gold, and many more.

I wanted to make it myself. In high school and college I had some chemistry training, I was also adept at vegan nutrition having started the first gourmet raw food restaurant in the United States. I had some experience. Most importantly I knew gold was inert in the body, so it was safe to experiment with it and I could be my own guinea pig in attempting to make it myself and get high off my own supply.

Even though science teaches that gold has no chemical reaction, now I was initiated into a higher awareness, the knowledge that in its reduced, altered, non-metallic form, gold is perhaps one of the most extraordinary healing agents ever discovered. This wasn't some magic fairy dust and wishful thinking, I can trust what I experienced; there was really something profound to this stuff.

I met and pondered with other enthusiasts, asking that age old question, "what is it?" I set out to learn everything I could about what I would refer to from then on as ORMUS Gold. ORMUS stands for Orbitally-Rearranged-Metal-Under-Study. David Hudson may have invented the term, I do not know. There was much to learn, and a lot of what I discovered, I believe only a handful of people on this planet are blessed with this knowledge. But the greater blessing is to share it with you, to give it to everyone that wants to try. Psst, hey. Here's a little gold kid, it won't hurt you.

In 2004 I travelled to India for half a year and discovered in their ancient lore and even recent medicinal practice, they know the power of healing with reduced potable gold quite well. In 2005, I networked into a small research group of scientists and laymen keen on unlocking the secrets of this "white gold". After three years of a lot of work, a good amount of trial and error and some dumb luck, we perfected a formula for what eventually became ORMUS GOLD®.

I really do consider this a whole and complete boon for humanity, such a small innocuous thing, yet extraordinary in its healing ability and a true panacea for optimum health; a real win-win unlike anything else. My work in our group centered on ceaseless research, further study and the practice of esoteric chemistry, and endeavoring to decode ancient formulas that had been written down through the ages. Using the conveniences of modern science, superior equipment, the help of a chemistry savant, a little blind luck and a whole bunch of pain and suffering, in a few years we pretty much figured it out. We had an ORMUS of gold that we could quantify and measure the potency, our highest yield of over 4% i.e., the amount of metallic gold converted to ORMUS from a starting material of 21 grams.

After a while, the riddles and vague instructions in the medieval alchemical books began to make sense. We cracked the formula, at least the first part, (the second part has to do with isolating the ORMUS in a pure state in which it behaves more like a gas). I believe we actually improved upon the purity of the gold medicines of the past as they did not have the high standards of modern chemistry or the knowledge we have today when it comes to mole ratios, the quality of lab equipment such as glass, high precision scales, and other tools as simple as a thermometer or as complex to make purified de-ionized 18 megohm water.

We invented a way to not only standardize and improve the "Philosopher's Stone" but drastically shorten the time to make it, while at the same time increasing the yield, along with the ability to quantify the exact percentage of monatomic gold in solution. Like all great discoveries of the past forty years, despite having the best equipment, it too was invented in a converted garage.

As rapid advancements occur in the fields of science and technology, many things hidden for a long time are now becoming known. Allow me to welcome you to the amazing catalytic health benefits of Gold!

**-Victor Sagalovsky**

# Introduction

Gold is the most coveted element on the planet and may very well be the missing trace mineral in our health. Gold is chemically inert it, so it is very safe to use in many biologically formats. It does not corrode. It is uneffected by moisture, oxygen or ordinary acids. It is one of the most efficient conductors of electricity. Its density enables it to be seen under electron microscopes. And though virtually indestructible, it is a soft metal, easy to work with, shape, flatten or draw out into microscopic strands. In the body, it works in ways science is yet discovering. Foremost it is a catalyst to activate and enhance many of the functions of the body.

It would reason to think that our bodies which also conduct electricity, aka life-force would benefit from supplementation with gold. And it does! However, the human body is not made from spare parts; not everything ingested is of benefit, that is determined by our ability to break down and assimilate these building blocks into our cellular matrix.

This is where nano-science comes in. Our intestinal tract, our bio-terrain, every beneficial microbe living in our gut is beneficial is ever diligently working to break down and reduce everything that comes in so that it may be made small enough to pass through cell walls and be assimilated.

Unfortunately, we can not digest elements without an enzyme chaperone; we rely on plants and lithophilic (rock eating) microbes to do this for us, and so we eat the plants which provide us the needed minerals with an enzyme catalyst, attached to a carbon, that makes it organic and usable by us.

Unfortunately, our bodies do not have the ability to dissolve gold, thus the secret that has been passed down through the ages, that if we can pre-digest the gold externally, and make it small enough, down to a single atom, then yes, the body can use it for all kinds of reactions that raise the phase angle of our cells, which is simply an increase in conductivity, a decrease in resistance, and an expansion of total capacity of life-force that we can conduct.

Monatomic and reduced particle size, i.e. nano or ORMUS gold has the potential to be the Aspirin of the 21st century. Meaning that it should be in everyone's medicine cabinet as an essential supplement, the ultimate panacea, an extraordinary healing agent; and a true catalyst of radiant health.

## What is Gold?

Classical science teaches us that are three phases of matter. These are gases, liquids, and solids. But now there other states such as called plasma, Bose-Einstein condensates and liquid crystals. Some solids crystallize into a lattice structure called metals. What classical science does not teach us is that there is, in fact, another phase of matter called monatomic. These monatomic materials have ceramic-like properties.

Let's look at the textbook definition of gold. Gold is a transition group 1 element and exists in nature in two form; metallic gold and ionic gold salts.

Metallic gold known as colloidal gold exists from 1 nm-100 size particles. Coarse gold particles are over 100 nm size. Colloidal gold absorbs different wavelengths of light from 510 nm – 560 nm depending on particle size, smaller particles absorbing light of shorter wavelength.

Because nano-colloidal gold absorbs light at 520 nm (green light) and 450 nm (blue light). The color of the solution is the result obtained when the green and blue components of white light are removed. The color of the solution, therefore, represents a composite of all colors transmitted (i.e., not absorbed) by the particles. Spherical gold nanoparticles from 10-100 nanometers go from black to purple to reddish orange and exceeding 100nm yellow gold.

In the monatomic non-metallic state the solution of gold looks almost clear to a slight violet hue. Now let's look at the definition of non-metallic gold.

In 1995, a new state of matter was discovered called Bose-Einstein condensates, as predicted by Albert Einstein and Satyendra Nath Bose in the 1920's. These states of matter exist parallel to their respective elements on the periodic table, but exhibit much different non-metallic properties. Some have speculated that Bose-Einstein condensates exist somewhere between spirit and matter and exhibit superconducting properties. Room temperature superconductivity is the holy grail in science, it makes limitless energy and levitation within the realm of practical possibilities. It is humanity's destiny to discover this and based on what we are starting to understand about monatomics, Bose-Einstein Condensates, Hadronic Mechanics, and magnetism we are not far off.

# What Makes Gold Non-Metallic?

A metallic element is physically stable and is usually a good conductor of electricity and heat and is chemically active as evidenced by oxidation and corrosion. Unlike their metallic counterparts, monatomic atoms of the same element behave closer to a ceramic as they are poor conductors of electricity and heat and are inert chemically.

When Gold is a metal, it is ionic, The most common forms of ionic gold are oxidation levels I (monovalent) and III (trivalent). This means that the electron in the outer orbital of the gold atom seek to bond with other electrons in other gold atoms creating a metallic compound. But gold atoms in their pure monatomic Einstein-Bose Condensate state exist as non-ionic and non-valent.

What this means is that thirteenth electron which normally bonds to other gold atoms (valent), instead is actually sucked into a lower orbit thereby changing the entire atomic structure of the atom, as the center of gravity moves closer to the nucleus, the spin is increased, and if there is no perturbation from an external force then there is no decay in spin, and superconducting properties can be observed.

In the late 80's nuclear physicists discovered that the atoms of certain elements exist in micro-clusters, between two and several hundred atoms. Most of what are known as transition group metals in the center of the periodic chart can exist in a monatomic state. More than a few hundred atoms in a micro-cluster and they form into a lattice structure which give them the metallic properties for which they are known. Less than a few hundred micro-clustered atoms and these elements stop behaving like metals and take on more ceramic type properties. Monatomic atoms are not held in position by electron sharing as with classical metallic bonds and chemical reactions. With monatomic gold, the valence electron is not available for sharing, and gold, in its reduced monatomic state behaves very different than its metallic counterpart.

Because the atoms of monatomic elements are not held in a rigid lattice network, their physical characteristics are quite different from atoms which are locked into a electron sharing lattice. So, in the future elements will not only be identified by the number of protons and neutrons in their nucleus, but also how they bond to one another. These monatomic elements are an entirely new phase of matter previously unknown to modern chemistry because conventional analytical technology, which detects elements based on their shared valence electrons, is unable to detect these atoms, since there is no chemical pairing with monatomic elements.

Gold, and other transition elements, turns out have this second monatomic phase, something not detected by science until Bose-Einstein condensates were proven to exist. With no method readily available to test it, the ORMUS must first be converted back to metallic state and quantitatively tested for gold metal adding on estimated losses.

David Hudson, who is not a scientist, but who has researched these monatomic elements probably more than anyone on the planet states that these monatomic elements can behave as room temperature superconductors.

The room temperature superconductor is one of the holy grails of science, and the global scientific consensus is that no such element exists or has yet been invented. Yet, Hudson's statements are consistent with anecdotal information gleaned from medieval alchemical texts that state that their alchemical preparations had properties of levitation. In fact, one text claims that these alchemically altered elements could be made into red glass and that this glass levitates. Such glass was incorporated into stained glass windows in European cathedrals, which are there to this day, levitating glass hidden in plain site.

In our own laboratory experiments we confirmed another of interesting observation made by Hudson and others, namely that the specific gravity of monatomic elements is not stable. As the gold material "cures", we have observed a drop in weight that we can not explain. Nearly half of the starting weight of the transitioning gold simply disappears over a matter of three weeks, fluctuating like a sine wave until it 4/9th of the original weight is gone. Although 95% of our research has been with gold, we did experiment with other elements and in one such experiment with monatomic copper found that when heated, the material levitated. Unfortunately, for lack of keeping good lab notes at the time, a subsequent attempt to recreate the experiment were unsuccessful.

The word monatomic is kind of a misnomer, since monatoms still bond with their counterparts, only its not a chemical bond, i.e., non-valent. When gold monatoms bond, they do so through a mechanism similar to what is called a Cooper-pairing, a state which is responsible for superconductivity, part of the BCS theory, which won the Nobel Prize for physics in 1972. Here is quantum mechanics explanation of how it works. An electron in a metal normally behaves as a free particle.

The electron is repelled from other electrons because of their negative charge, while attracting positive ions which make up the lattice that creates the metallic form of the element. These ions become distorted because of the attractive force, which moves these ions toward the electron, which increases the density of the positive charge and attracts other electrons. The electrons form a bond because their repelling force is overcome by the displaced ions.

So it is the high-spin state of the gold monatoms that creates an attractive force, not the valent electrons, and so two monatoms pair up, and this is a Cooper pair. This type of energy pairing is quite weak. In the case of ORMUS gold, that means a strong electromagnetic force or positively or negatively charged ions will break the bond, and the monatoms will go back to their metallic state.

Monatomic elements, it is theorized, are responsible for the superconducting properties of all living things. This is because Cooper pairs have shown to be able to transfer energy from nucleus to nucleus without loss of energy. This is the state that is between pure matter and pure energy. It is believed that monatomic elements compose about 5% of the dry weight of the nervous system. Is this the 21 grams that mysteriously disappears upon the cessation of life?

Although there are a dozen metals that will effect a monatomic state, the reason I have focused on gold is it is the one that has proven itself to be the most beneficial for general physical healing and is the only one of the elements that is completely non-toxic in its pure form. The FDA and WHO/FAO consider gold as a safe additive to food and for external use.

Certainly I hope to experiment more with creating monatomics from other platinum group elements and especially Ruthenium which was shown in a experiment conducted in the early 90's and written about in the May 1995 issue of Scientific American to increase the conductivity of DNA by thousands of times when Ruthenium monatoms were placed on each end of the double helix, thus showing the complete lack of electrical resistance between the atoms. Lighter elements, like copper, that have no unoccupied orbital positions, are converted to ORMUS not by deactivating valence electrons, but by the application of megavolts of electrical power which spin these electrons to some unknown great distance away from the core of the copper atom, causing copper ORMUS to levitate when heated. But that is another story. For now, gold will remain the main subject of our interest because of the life giving properties inherent in its reduced state.

Natural ORMUS exists in small amounts in dark and undisturbed places often found and identified within ore samples, but they lack quantity needed to be signicant and unless refined always nor pure. The high-purity ORMUS elements, the U.S. department of Defense has classified as "strategic materials," mostly because of their implications within aerospace, robotics and energy production.

Unfortunately, there is a lot of misunderstanding when it comes to gold's role in physical health. Because gold has no chemical interactions in vivo, mistakenly it has been classified as inert with no recommended daily allowance as a trace element. But what is little understood is how it works as a catalyst aiding the transduction of bio-electrical signals to structured light, and vice-versa. A good example of structured light is DNA.

Here's a big bold statement: monatomic/high-spin state/non-valent gold is the most fractal substance in nature. What is a fractal? A fractal is a never-ending pattern. Fractals are infinitely complex patterns that are self-similar across different scales. So a fractal is able to compress itself without loss of information, to nest infinitely within itself. It is like a hologram, where every part contains the whole, and every smaller part is self similar to every larger part.

My theory is that this type of gold particle exists as a bridge between the third and fourth dimensions, between time and timelessness, translating inner light to electrical potential and vice-versa. Can I prove it? Not yet. Do a lot of people agree? Oh yes! Can this lead us to the holy grail of scientific discoveries, the room temperature superconductor? Yes, it will. The room temperature superconductor will usher in a new age for humanity, with no decay of spin many things become possible such as limitless clean energy, interstellar space travel, and the extension of lifespan. I think what is happening with ORMUS Gold is it enhances energy flow within the microtubules inside every living cell, which we will get into more detail later. Can this lead to physical immortality or at least the doubling or tripling of our current human life spans? To this question I offer a passage from The Golden Tract, an alchemical compendium of much earlier work, published in 1678:

"As for the Elixir of Life, conferring immortality is the prerogative of God alone, but to quote from an old book: By virtue of this quintessence, Artephius testifieth that he lived above a thousand years; Flamel also recordeth it, that it triumpeth over all the miseries of the world, Laznioro is more bold, and saith, that if in the agonies of death, a man should taste but a grain of it, all mortal pestilence would depart from him."

If we are to believe in atomic transmutation, that in our very own cells certain elements can atomically transmutate to other elements, as has been proven by Kervran, Kamaki and so many other scientists, then its an interesting and important observation to know that the only two times gold is found in human tissue naturally is in mothers milk, (Trace Elements in Human Breast Milk. R.M. Parr IAEA Bulletin), as well as semen. A small amount of gold in the breast milk is transferred to the newborn for what purpose? Why is it present in semen? Does it have something to do with jump starting superconductivity in the embryo and the newborn?

Medieval alchemists referred to these monatomics as prima matria (first matter), and aurum potabile (gold elixir). They were very clear that these elements are very different from their metallic forms.

Many researchers I have been in contact with have identified these materials in this alternate phase of matter. They have arrived at many of the same observations, that these nano particle orbitally rearranged elements exhibit superconductivity, superfluidity, and Josephson tunneling meaning they can resist magnetic fields and levitate. In our research we have found these non-valent atoms exist in this Cooper paired monatomic state as long as they are not disturbed by external electrons. Once energy is introduced, this exotic matter is displaced out of its high spin state and becomes covalent once again.

Let's look at a theory of how ORMUS Gold works. Gold itself possesses a property of being an excellent reflector of near infrared radiations (NIR). Cells transmit, receive, and act upon signals of near infrared in predictable manners. Gold with small particle sizes of less than 10 nm could act as a wide angle diffuser of near infrared signals. Since spatial coherence of electromagnetic signals is required for cellular recognition, wide angle diffusers favor spatial coherence of near infrared signals by reaching the whole circumference of neighboring cells at the same time. So gold its reduced form may actually improve cellular communication by making the signaling more efficient. If this is a fact then the intercellular exchange of information between the cytoplasm and the nucleus of the cell should increase, thereby increasing RNA synthesis. This catalytic stimulating effect, particularly as seen in its ability to increase production of collagen and elastin explains this rejuvenating property.

## GOLD + SILICA = AUROSILICA

In nature, gold is often found bound to silica, and without it we wouldn't be able to make ORMUS gold. Silica provides stability to monatomic Cooper-paired gold atoms, keeping them from bonding back to one another to make metallic gold. ORMUS Gold exists as non-valent held in a matrix of Silica.

If it were to be removed from the silica, the ORMUS Gold might actually be more like a gas and evaporate readily at room temperature. This is written about in the medieval alchemical texts, one particular passage being when the alchemist St. Germaine offers a vial to a curious observer and says to be very careful in opening it because it can easily escape. Thus, ORMUS Gold is created and sustained by the assistance of pure silica.

Nobel Prize winner (1993) Professor Adolf Butenandt proved silica to be an essential mineral to sustain life. The typical human body holds roughly seven grams of silica, much more than most other key minerals. Silica is essential to the metabolic processes that are vital to life. As we age, predictably, the source of silica in our bodies becomes exhausted, resulting in all kinds of degenerative and aging issues.

Silica has been regarded as nature's building block and is our answer to healthier, younger looking, more radiant skin, hair and nails. It is a universal element in the human body that can be found free and soluble in water or combined with proteins and lipids, and has an exact relationship to mineral absorption. Its most important purpose is of immune nature, because the Silica partakes in the manufacturing process of antibodies/antigens and it encourages the conversion of Lymphocyte B into Lymphocyte T.

So when ingesting ORMUS Gold, one not only gets the benefit of the gold, but also the silica, which is made bioavailable by its reduced size and solubility in water at a neutral pH which has not has not been observed in organic chemistry before. Normally Silicic acid only goes soluble, but in the case of ORMUS Gold®, the orthosilica goes soluble in a completely non-ionic medium.

What happens, in theory, is when the monatomic gold is 'curing', i.e., the gold bonds are breaking, and the valence electron of the monatomic gold atoms are pulled into a lower orbit. The polar bond angle of the hydrogen in water, which is normally 104.5 degrees, compresses, pushing the hydrogen atoms closer together. I believe this to be the reason silica goes soluble at a neutral pH.

When energy is added back into the system the monatomic gold will go back to metallic. When this happens, the silica falls out of solution and becomes gel again. My belief with the topical use of monatomic gold is as such; sometimes the silica absorbs and sometimes it is left behind as a dry white residue, indication that the monatomic gold has absorbed. This can be attributes this to the bodies innate management system, if silica is lacking, it goes in, as it is after all bio-available, and if silica is not lacking then it stay behind. You can say that's weird but that is my qualitative observation.

# REAL GOLD ORMUS VS. FAKE

Let's set the record straight, as the internet is rife with products purporting to be monatomic gold, when in reality, most of the products this author has tested contain no monatomic gold or any gold whatsoever. How can one know what is a true monatomic healing therapeutic?

Here are some clues. If there is anything else in the ingredients list other than gold, then run away. Monatomic gold can only exist by itself, in a pH neutral environment. If there are any spare electrons of anything in the solution, it will quickly agitate the monatoms of gold out of their high-spin state and the solution will start the chain reaction of converting back to larger clusters of metallic gold.

Colloidal gold has plenty of benefit, but it is not monatomic. Next, if the alleged monatomic gold is made from seawater or a natural earthen deposit, chances are there is more in it than just gold. In nature, gold, as we know, is never alone, so trace amounts of other heavy metals will be present. We derive no benefit from ingesting elements in their metallic state. If we did, we would be able to eat rocks and forego the need for plants. Many self styled alchemists have perished from ingesting material that they believed was doing them benefit but in fact was full of heavy metals and metallic salts bringing much harm to the organs and central nervous system. As we must know and purify ourselves, we must know to purify anything that it is not organic and that is easily absorbs into the blood and the brain. The number one rule of life is to not bring harm to self. And as they say, a little knowledge is a dangerous thing.

# How We Make It

The formula we created is not much different from the ancients, at least that's what we've been able to discern from the historical literature about the making of it.

I've listed all the old alchemy books I have investigated at the end of this book; they are not easy to find, but some of them have been archived online. What we're simply doing is taking gold, in this case we start with a Canadian Gold dollar which is minted by Johnson-Mathey, the purest gold available at 99.99%.

We refine it further, to 99.9999%. That takes quite a few steps and lots of time. We have tried making the ORMUS with 99.99%, but if there are any atoms of any other metal in there, you won't get any ORMUS. What we have after our gold refinement is something at the bottom of the glass that is the most a rich ruby red liquid.

This is converted to a golden yellow powder sometimes called auric acid, a monatom of gold connected to a hydroxide (OH-). Now you have a worthy starting material. 500 year old alchemy books describe this process within their cryptic instructions. If you made it right, what you now essentially have is gold atoms that have dropped their metallic bonds and are now only bound to OH-, one of the most widely studied, and most beneficial antioxidants in nature, found in water, food and everything life giving. But we have to break that bond and have the individual gold monatoms detach from their trivalent bond and go from Gold III to Gold 0. We do a simple process that was incredibly painstaking to create, and this is why in the medieval alchemy books it was called "drudgery and women's work." Unfortunately, they weren't exactly egalitarian.

What gives our method near perfect repeatability and improves on the ancient techniques of purification is we know the atomic weight of gold is 196.967g. This weight in grams is called a gram atom. Likewise oxygen has an atomic weight of 16. It is written as $O_2$ because it is diatomic as a gas under normal atmosphere conditions. Thus 16 x 2 = 32 grams. This weight in grams is called a gram mole. The gram mole carries exactly the same number of molecules as does the gram atom carry atoms. This is true of all elements and compounds made up of various elements, this magic number is called Avogadro's Constant. Again, it is the total number of atoms or molecules in a gram mole or gram atom of anything. This number is 602,2xx,xx0,000,000,000,000,000. Fifth to eighth places, marked with x's, have been varied attempting to make the constant more accurate ever since 1810. The fifth place is less than .001% of the total, so all changes have made very little difference in the "big picture." Avogadro's Constant is more easily written as scientific notation: $6.022xxxx \times 10^{23}$.

What we do is force each gold atom to drop its bond with the OH-. Atoms locked by shared electrons are released of their attachments. And over time gold falls off. As it does the valence shell, that free 13th electron constantly wanting to pair with another gold or just about any other atom, as we theorize, gets sucked into a lower orbit, displacing the atomic structure of the atom. Now it is no longer metallic gold at all.

Now it is something else entirely, a different element, an exotic state of matter, something that is against its very nature. Let me make an analogy to illustrate. Imagine taking a highly animalistic procreativity focused creature and removing its desire for anything external so it can sit for many days in pure and complete stillness, in a trance that can only occur if one is not disturbed. That means getting bombarded by whatever electrons or cosmic rays are needed to wake it up and make it pop that lone electron looking to go out on the town and get into trouble back to its lonely position in the 13th shell.

So if you want that gold to drop and go monatomic, the key is that you remove all energy from the environment. It is the most perfect meditation, the transformation that happens is really Zen, pure stillness, zero effort, the letting go, releasing at the subatomic level. And then going with the flow.

Once the atom releases and goes into its zero-valent state, it does go into a faster spin, faster at the core, but now its other orbitals elongated. Because we haven't been able to observe it with a microscope yet, we theorize the atom goes from .8 to 1.2 Angstrom in size.

When you have many of these monatomic gold atoms, they do have a type of attractive force, even though they are non-valent, and they lock in and spin together with other gold monatoms. This I have explained as Cooper pairing.

Now you have these monatoms and Cooper pairs, and if they weren't in a soluble silica, they would fly away like a gas. The silica keeps this alchemical gold stable. It is only a glass castle, so although it appears strong, it is easily broken. The main reaction and days of purification steps all have to be done in a completely EMF shielded environment, when no moon or sun are present in the sky. It is done under darkness, where there is absolutely no outside force or vector of excitation, be it electron, x-ray, EMF or any wave that could disturb the necessary stillness of this meditation.

ORMUS GOLD® is adjusted to a concentration of 5 mg per fluid ounce. The concentration of product out of an average yield reaction is most often close to this or slightly higher. When all the "did not take in the reaction" gold is reclaimed from the extensive water washes and is compared to the total gold used in the beginning of the ORMUS preparation sequence, the amount that did take is easily and accurately calculated, then precisely adjusted by adding the proper amount of deoxygenated deionized water. After this is done, the curing takes place which is the event that creates the ORMUS. During this last curing stage, gold slowly yet steadily dissociated from its silica chain carriers and in a purely non-ionic low energy environment the valence shells become orbitally rearranged, the liquid goes from cloudy white to clear and we have ORMUS. The leftover silica chains become soluble silicic acid, $H_2SiO_3$. It will remain as such, in a clarified state so long as ORMUS gold remains within the matrix. When the $Au^0$ reverts back to $Au^1$, the cloudy silica gel chains begin to reappear. Expensive analytical conditional determinations are never needed, only the clarity of the solution let's you know if there's ORMUS in the bottle. 5 mg of ORMUS per ounce doesn't sound much, which when you do the math is $1.528 \times 10^{19}$. Quintillions of ORMUS gold atoms.

## Historical Uses

The earliest records of the use of gold for medicinal and healing purposes come from Alexandria, Egypt. Over 5,000 years ago, the Egyptians ingested gold for mental, bodily and spiritual purification. The ancients believed that gold in the body worked by stimulating the life force and raising the level of vibration on all levels.

The Alchemists of Alexandria developed an "elixir" made of liquid gold. They believed that gold was a mystical metal that represented the perfection of matter, and that its presence in the body would enliven, rejuvenate, and cure a multitude of diseases as well as restore youth and perfect health. As long as 4,500 years ago, the Egyptians also used gold in dentistry. Remarkable examples of gold's early use has been found by modern archaeologists.

Still in favor today as an ideal material for dental work, approximately 15 tons of gold are used each year for crowns, bridges, inlays and dentures. Gold is ideal for these purposes because it is non-toxic, can be shaped easily, and never wears, corrodes or tarnishes. In short, it is the most perfect metal there is.

Mahdihassan, a notable historian on alchemy, claimed that the Chinese were the first to prepare and use reduced gold as the alchemical drug of longevity, but he gave no reference. According to Mahdihassan, the word alchemy derives from two Chinese words: "Kim" (gold) and "Yeh" (juice). "Kimyeh" (gold juice) entered the Arabic language as "kimiya", and with the definite article, "al," the Arabic word for ingestible gold was "alkimiya," which in the western world gave the word "alchemy". So alchemy means preparation and use of potable gold.

Alchemy and the use of gold supplements spread from China to Arabia and then throughout the Middle East to India and eventually Europe. Even today in China, the belief in the restorative properties of gold remain intact in rural villages, where peasants cook their rice with a gold coin to replenish the gold in their bodies and fancy Chinese restaurants put 24-karat gold-leaf in their food preparations.

It was reported that in the early 1900's doctors would implant a $5.00 gold piece near a knee joint to help with arthritis. Since 1927, gold salts have been used to relieve joint discomfort and damage in the United States. Europeans have long been aware of the benefits of gold in the body and have been buying gold coated pills and 'gold water' over the counter for well over 300 years.

Today, gold netting is used in surgery to patch damaged blood vessels, nerves, bones, and membranes. Modern physicians inject microscopic gold to help retard prostate cancer in men and women with ovarian cancer are treated with gold solutions. Gold vapor lasers seek out and destroy cancerous cells without harming their healthy neighbors and give new life to patients with once inoperable heart conditions and tumors.

One experimental new gold compound blocks virus replication in infected cells and is being tested for the treatment of AIDS. By attaching a molecular marker to a microscopic piece of gold, called tracing, scientists can follow its movement through the body. Some researchers are placing gold on DNA to study the hybrid genetic material in cells, while others are using it to determine how cells respond to toxins, heat and physical stress. Because it is biologically benign and easy to trace, biochemists use gold to form compounds with proteins to create new lifesaving drugs. Gold is truly the perfection of the metals.

Saint Hildegard of Bingen (1098-1179), Patron of National Guild of Water Diviners and Bioenergy Therapists recommended and used various gold treatments. She highly recommended baking powdered gold with spelt flour and water and drinking wine with gold. She claimed that gold taken regularly, even in very small doses, is an essential element for human body, even though it occurs in trace amounts. Hildegard recommended using gold for all physical and mental problems.

According to her, gold was not only the symbol of purity but also longevity, developed mental and moral features, and was an all around excellent elixir for health. The great alchemist, and father of Pharmacology, Paracelsus (1493-1541) who first prepared nano gold solution in modern times. He called his solution of gold Aurum Potabile and believed it cured all manner of physical, mental, and spiritual ailments.

"Gold receives its influence from the Sun," he wrote: "which is, as it were, the Heart of the world and by communicating these influences to the human heart it serves to fortify and cleanse it from all impurities."

The alchemists believed that gold represented the perfection of matter, and that its presence in the body would enliven, rejuvenate, and cure a multitude of disturbances in the life force. The alchemists believed this type of exotic gold had a balancing and harmonizing effect on all levels of body, mind, and spirit.

It was used to improve mental attitude and treat unstable mental and emotional states such as depression, melancholy, sorrow, fear, despair, anguish, frustration, suicidal tendencies, seasonal effective disorder, poor memory, poor concentration, and many other imbalances in mind, body, and spirit. Angelo Sala, a Venetian philosopher and alchemist who lived in 16th century was known for successfully using gold saline against measles and water dropsy.

After studying the work of Paracelsus, the English scientist Michael Faraday prepared nano gold in 1857, and many uses were found for his solutions of "activated gold." In 1890, the distinguished German bacteriologist Robert Koch won the Nobel Prize for his discovery that compounds made with gold inhibited growth of bacteria. Edgar Cayce the twentieth century's most famous American psychic and mystic believed the balance of elements in the human body is disturbed by a shortage of gold. In his readings he claimed that gold was essential in the workings of all glands. He believed it was helpful in the treatment of cancer, rheumatism, inflammation of lymph, multiple sclerosis, thyroid conditions, Alzheimer's and Parkinson's, alcoholism, mental illnesses, menopause, and infertility.

The procedure for the preparation of potable gold by comminution is still in use today in India, prescribed by Ayurvedic physicians for rejuvenation and revitalization in old age under the name "Swarna Bhasma" (red gold), with a reputation of being extremely safe. Granules of metallic gold are placed in a granite mortar, mixed with some herbal extracts and rubbed with a granite pestle until the mixture develops a brick red color, a procedure requiring two months.

The red orange color suggests that the particles are quite small, less than 20 nm. Although this was not monatomic gold, which is much more finer, it was an effective, albeit crude preparation. Unfortunately, we also know some Ayurvedic physicians wanted the color of their reduced gold to be blood red, so they added red mercury sulfide (cinnabar) to the gold colloids. This made the medicine very toxic and may be the reason Swarna Basma went into disrepute in recent times. However, Bajaj and Vahora commented that reduced gold was still popular in India (as of 1998) and is "highly valued for its tonic and rejuvenating properties." According to these investigators, ayurvedic physicians recommend swarna bhasma as a general tonic, hepato tonic, cardio tonic, nervine tonic, aphrodisiac, detoxicant, anti-infective, with anti-aging benefit.

## Modern Uses

Today, medical uses of gold have expanded greatly. From orthopedics to cancer, and new medical research coming out every year, gold is on positive track in modern medicine.

Gold is currently used in surgery to patch damaged blood vessels, nerves, bones, and membranes. It is also used in the treatment of several forms of cancer. Injection of microscopic gold pellets helps retard prostate cancer in men. Women with ovarian cancer are treated with colloidal gold, and gold vapor lasers help seek out and destroy cancerous cells without harming their healthy neighbors. Everyday, surgeons use gold instruments to clear coronary arteries, and gold-coated lasers give new life to patients with once inoperable heart conditions and tumors.

Gold has become an important biomedical tool for scientists studying why the body behaves as it does. By attaching a molecular marker to a microscopic piece of gold, scientists can follow its movement through the body. Because gold is readily visible under an electron microscope, scientists can now actually observe reactions in individual cells.

Reduced nano gold is known for its powers as an anti-inflammatory and is reputed to be a powerful glandular rejuvenate with life extension, raised brain function and I.Q. and pineal enhancing possibilities. (Frontier Perspectives, Vol 7, No 2, Fall 1998). Doctors Cairo and Brinckmann wrote a best selling work in the early 60's in Brazil entitled "Materia Medica", in which they claimed, based on their own clinical experience that potable gold was their preferred go-to remedy for obesity.

Gold preparations have also been known to be effective for easing the pains and swellings of arthritis, rheumatism, bursitis, and tendonitis. Gold compounds have historically been used in drugs for the treatment of a wide range of ailments. This use of gold compounds in medicine is called chrysotherapy.

The Frenchman Jacques Forestier reported in 1929 that the use of gold complexes was beneficial in the treatment of arthritis. Later work after the Second World War demonstrated conclusively that gold drugs are effective in treating rheumatoid arthritis patients. Two of the most commonly referred to gold compounds in such treatments are Myocrisin and Auranofin. In July 1935, the medical periodical "Clinical, Medicine & Surgery" had an article entitled "Colloidal Gold in Inoperable Cancer" written by Edward H. Ochsner, M.D., Chicago-Consulting Surgeon, Augustana Hospital. He stated,

"When the condition is hopeless, Colloidal Gold helps prolong life and makes life much more bearable, both to the patient and to those about them, because it shortens the period of terminal cachexia (general physical wasting and malnutrition usually associated with chronic disease) and greatly reduces pain and discomfort and the need of opiates (narcotics) in a majority of instances."

Gold possesses a high degree of resistance to bacterial colonization and because of this it is the material of choice for implants that are at risk of infection, such as the inner ear. Gold has a long tradition of use in this application and is considered a very valuable metal in microsurgery of the ear. The isotope gold-198, (half-life: 2.7 days) is used in some cancer treatments and for treating other diseases. It should also be noted that without gold's reliability for electronic components within medical devices such as pacemakers and ventilators, many medical treatments would not be as effective as they are today.

An official U.S. study on gold therapy in human subjects involved the orally active aurothiolate Auranofin (Ridaura) from Smith, Kline, and French. There was no evidence of toxicity of this colloidal metallic gold at the clinical, histological cellular and molecular levels. They concluded that their gold based pharmaceutical with a size in the low nanometer range is a safe and effective alternative to the toxic aurothiolates in the management of rheumatoid arthritis and tuberculosis.

In a study with the elderly, nano gold in tablet form (Aurasol®) at a daily intake of 20 mg for eight weeks was evaluated using various parameters assessed by procedures previously validated. The design was double-blind longitudinal, non-crossover, using grape juice extract in the placebo tablets to give the same appearance as the colloidal gold tablets. This just means that one group got the gold, the other group got the placebo, and no one knew which they got.

Not surprisingly, there was no beneficial effect in the elderly receiving placebo tablets. However, in the subjects on colloidal gold, there was significant improvement of overall well-being, coordination, equilibrium, pain, energy level, cognition, physical well being, and short-term memory.

Whether an essential element or not, nano particulate gold may be useful on a long-term basis in the elderly and on everyone for that matter because of the beneficial effect on mental and physical well-being.

In Homeopathy gold is also considered an important healing therapeutic. Aurum metallicum is prescribed for deep depression and suicidal states. Ingestion of this homeopathic stimulates an improvement in self esteem and self worth. Feelings of isolation, joylessness, anorexia nervosa and chronic fatigue are addressed with the use of this remedy.

As mentioned previously, what I have observed in the making of ORMUS Gold is that the water molecule that is part of the ORMUS is altered. The water bound to the gold monatoms seems to act more like heavy water, (deuterium). I have not been able to quantify this hypothesis yet but I do believe the polar bond angle of the two hydrogen atoms is pulled closer together. Is it the high spin state of the potentially Cooper paired monatoms creating a force that pulls the bond angle of water tighter?

In the field of chemistry and nano-material science this is an important discovery, made in a garage lab with no Ph.D scientists on staff!

This observed restructuring of water is quite significant and also may serve as the basis of Homeopathy as first proposed by Rustum Roy. I believe this fundamental alteration is a key to contributor to what makes this "Celestial Water" significant for health, as it energizes the morphogenic field of the body, increasing the speed of intra- and intercellular communications.

Since gold is an excellent conductor of electricity, it acts as a sub-cellular semiconductor, capacitor and its most rarefied form a superconductor. Superconducting means no decay of spin, no resistance, perpetual effortless motion, not effected by gravity.

Intracellularly reduced nano gold would increase not only the amount of information exchanged between cells within subcellular organelles but also would increase the speed of this transfer of information. Such mechanisms could explain the improved cognitive functions following nano gold ingestion.

Could it be that the mechanism we are dealing with here is intelligent structured light. Ultraviolet and infrared signaling is our cells all the way down to the DNA communicate. Light is the language of life and gold is the conductor. Furthermore, Japanese researchers found that gold clusters below 10nm elicited a protective immune response in mice inoculated with plasmids encoding Japanese encephalitis virus. These nano gold particles Small adsorb on the Fc portion of IgG antibodies leaving the FAB active sites more available for binding to antigens. This stabilizing effect of gold colloids on IgG antibodies could improve immune functions and increase resistance to infections.

For many centuries the Indian system of medicine known as Ayurveda mentions the role of gold in the treatment of male infertility. 'Swarna Bhasma' (Ash of gold) has been used with good results by Ayurvedic practitioners in the treatment of infertility. Hence, a study was planned to estimate gold in whole semen by atomic absorption spectrophotometry. Whole semen from 11 healthy and fertile males was analyzed for gold content by Atomic Absorption spectrophotometry. On analysis all semen samples were found to contain gold ranging from 0.36 to 1.98 μg/ml with a mean value of 0.88 μg/ml and a standard deviation of 0.51 μg/ml. In this study, gold was estimated after complete digestion (oxidation of organic matters; hence, whatever amount of gold detected, denotes the levels in seminal plasma as well as the sperm itself) in whole semen (seminal plasma and sperm).

It seems that the hypothesis made for presence of gold in sperm may be true. However, little prior literature is available on this and further studies are needed for scientific documentation of gold in male infertility.

# A Review of Benefits

The benefits of gold therapy are simply profound. With all the conditions it helps to treat, and the inability to patent a natural substance, no wonder it has not received the attention it deserves from the pharmaceutical obsessed medical world. Among other uses, monatomic gold can also be used as an aphrodisiac, and to quell the cravings for alcohol, and has been used as a remedy for digestive disorders, circulatory problems, depression, obesity, and burns. Gold can have a balancing and harmonizing effect on the body particularly with regard to unstable mental and emotional states, such as depression, S.A.D. (Seasonal effective Disorder), melancholy, sorrow, fear, despair, anguish, frustration, suicidal tendencies; the maladies commonly referred to as the "sicknesses of the heart".

Gold has been known down through the ages to have a direct effect on the activities of the heart, helping to improve blood circulation. It is known to be beneficial for rejuvenating sluggish organs, especially the digestive system (constipation) and brain. Gold has been used in cases of glandular and nervous incoordination, helping to rejuvenate the glands, stimulate the nerves and release nervous pressure.

The body's warmth mechanism may be positively effected by gold, particularly in cases of chills, hot flashes, night sweats and menopausal symptoms. A daily combination of silver and gold monatomic water appears to support our bodies natural defense system against disease and help promote renewed vitality and longevity. Monatomic gold assists to improve natural immunity and vitality, it has got positive influence on balancing the heart's pulse and circulation of the blood. Monatomic gold does not cause any irritation or addiction.

Monatomic gold influences both physical and emotional conditions. Gold therapy stabilizes collagen. It rejuvenates the brain, making one feel younger, it supports the digestive system, improves overall vitality and helps to regulate body temperature, improving and stimulating glands and the nervous system. It liquidates effects of allergy. Monatomic gold is also anti-acne. It supports treatment of: alcoholism, drug addiction, obesity, digestive problems, glandular hyperfunction, neurosis, depression, anxiety. It supports proper brain functions. It makes burns and cuts heal better, it alleviates muscles pain, excessive sweating as well as hot flashes and shivering. It also does not interact with any drugs. Monatomic gold can also help to regulate body temperature. Gold is a catalyst for endorphin-like hormones, as well as the antioxidant enzyme SOD, which neutralizes the negative effects of superoxide, a powerful oxidizer our bodies use to fend off pathogens, but which without SOD would compromise our bodies as well.

People with gold allergies are usually reacting to the other base metals added to gold jewelry such as nickel, copper, tin and even silver. The addition of these metals makes the gold easier to work with while at the same time increases durability. In each instance, we are talking about coarse metallic gold, not the bioactive colloidal or monatomic forms. Unlike colloidal silver (argyria) the internal consumption of gold has no known side effects or toxicity. Ionic gold known as gold chloride is also used in medicine, especially in the treatment of rheumatoid arthritis, but this type of gold is not recommended because it is in the form of a chloride, so it can be toxic if ingested.

Let's look at all the historical and modern uses of gold therapy in alphabetical order:

Alcoholism, Allergies, Alzheimer's (memory loss), Arthritis (forms including Rheumatoid), Asthma, Blood Circulation, Blood Pressure control & assists relaxation, Body Temperature Stabilizer, Brain Benefits, Brain: increases IQ by up to 35% (based on scientific study), Bruxism (teeth grinding), Bursitis (Inflammation), Crohn's Disease, Concentration & Focus, Coordination Aid, Dementia, Dependencies Reducer: Cigarettes, Drugs, etc., Depression: helps & prevents – excellent for depression, Diabetes, Discs: aids ruptured, swollen & slipped, Digestive System & Aid, Diverticulitis (inflammation of the diverticulum), Emotional Health Benefit & Balances, Eyesight, Frustration, Sorrow, Fear, Despair, Anguish, Gland stimulator, Gout, Heart Conditions, Heart: Regulates pumping rhythm, High Cholesterol, Hyperactivity, Insomnia, Joint Stiffness: due to degenerative conditions, Melancholy, Memory Aid, Mental Focus Benefit, Mental Function Benefit, Mental State Benefit, Motor Skills, Muscles: relieves pain of Pulled Muscle, Nerve Damage (Neuropathy), Nervous Congestion Aid, Osteoporosis: Fights, Pain Reducer, Physical Health Benefiter, Purification – Bodily, Purification – Mental, Restless Leg Syndrome, Skin Ulcers: accelerates healing, Suicidal tendencies, Seasonal effective Disorder (S.A.D.), Tendon Regeneration, Tuberculosis, Tumor Treatment, Ulcerative Colitis, Ulcers.

# THE HARVARD STUDY

In 1890, a German doctor named Robert Koch found that gold effectively killed the bacteria that caused tuberculosis. In the 1930s, based on a widely held but probably erroneous connection at the time between tuberculosis and rheumatoid arthritis, a French doctor, Jacques Forestier, developed the use of gold drugs for the treatment of rheumatoid arthritis. Gold drugs have been used since then as an effective treatment for this and other autoimmune diseases such as Lupus, but treatment can take months for action and sometimes presents severe side effects which have diminished their use in recent years.

Rheumatoid arthritis and other autoimmune diseases have been treated with gold preparations since the turn of the 20th century. In the February 2006 issue of Nature Chemical Biology Harvard Medical School researchers reported that a possible mode of action for the efficacy of these gold compounds was discovered. Brian DeDecker, PhD of the Department of Cell Biology at Harvard, the lead author of the study said: "We were searching for a new drug to treat autoimmune diseases, but instead we discovered a biochemical mechanism that may help explain how an old drug works." DeDecker and co-author Stephen De Wall, PhD., undertook a large-scale search for new drugs that would suppress the function of an important component of the immune system, MHC class II proteins, which are associated with autoimmune diseases. MHC class II proteins normally hold pieces of invading bacteria and virus on the surface of specialized antigen presenting cells. Presentation of these pieces alerts other specialized recognition cells of the immune system called lymphocytes, which starts the normal immune response.

Usually this response is limited to harmful bacteria and viruses, but sometimes this process goes awry and the immune system turns towards the body itself causing autoimmune diseases such as juvenile diabetes, Lupus, and rheumatoid arthritis. During their search through thousands of compounds they found that the known cancer drug, Cisplatin, a drug containing the metal platinum, directly stripped foreign molecules from the MHC class II protein.

From there, they found that platinum was just one member of a class of metals, including a special form of gold, that all render MHC class II proteins inactive. In subsequent experiments in cell culture, gold compounds were shown to render the immune system antigen presenting cells inactive. The cardiotonic effect of gold nano compounds could be due to the smaller particles (less than 6 nm) which are able to penetrate inside the mitochondria and nucleus of the cardiac myocytes.

Salnikov, et al, reported in 2007, that in isolated rat ventricular myocytes, only gold nano-colloids of 3-nm diameter could penetrate inside the nucleus and the mitochondria whereas particles of 6 nm could cross the cell membrane and concentrate in the cytosol but not in the mitochondria and nucleus of ventricular myocytes. The effect of small gold particles on mitochondrial synthesis of ATP could explain their cardiotonic effect.

## Skin Rejuvenation

There's been a lot of talk recently about the use of gold masks in spas. Well, one thing is there is a lot of bad and erroneous information. Those Gold masks people put on their face simply do not work effectively.

The gold particles are not small enough to be absorbed and utilized by your body. True, some gold ions get in under the pores and do their magic, but the price to benefit ratio is simply not there. Cleopatra is reported to have undergone a procedure similar to one currently being offered by various plastic surgeons.

Tiny gold nano-wires are inserted under the skin of the face and over a six month period the gold ions slowly released into the skin to combat wrinkles. But this is extreme. All you need for the same effect is gold in a nano state which will absorb into the epidermis and help restore collagen and elastin much easier, no plastic surgeons needed. In ancient Rome, gold salves were used for the treatment of disfiguring skin lesions and ulcers. Were these an ORMUS of gold perhaps?

Today, gold leaf plays an important role in the treatment of chronic skin ulcers. Gold and skin have a long story together. This is because it assists to stimulate collagen production and that leads to a myriad of benefits.

These are the traditional ones for external use that I collected from published literature, testimonials, and personal experience:

- To exhibit antiseptic and anti-inflammatory properties.

- To help cuts heal better.

- To enhance ionic movement in tissues to improve circulation.

- To reduce fine lines and wrinkles.

- To improve the firmness and elasticity of the skin.

- To tighten pores and smooth the skin.

- To hydrate skin from losing moisture.

- To help increase nutrients into the skin.

- To regenerate cells.

- To vitalize skin metabolism.

- To synergize the absorption of collagen, nutrients and essences of herbal and botanical extracts.

- To regulate or balance oil/fat secretion to protect the skin from bacteria.

- To delay the aging process.

# How to Use on Skin

This is the instructions for using ORMUS Gold, (the product we make), which in my observation has remarkable benefits for the skin. If your pores are closed, the gold won't get in, so keep that of the highest importance. Your face hands and skin must be freshly washed, with soap, and free of dirt and oil, as these act as a barrier preventing gold's absorption.

The skin, when the pores are open, absorbs the monatomic particles of gold where the catalyzing properties begin to take effect. Squeeze a full dropper of ORMUS in your cupped hand and rub onto face or massage into body.

For specific areas of concern, apply carefully by the drop, and let it dry and absorb. It is best to repeat this process twice during the same period for targeted areas, and then when it dries and a silica film remains upon the second application, wipe or wash it off, and you can add a nice skin oil on, one rich in squalene and beneficial lipids. Normally, some silica will absorb and some will stay behind.

This author believes the silica is bioavailable. Drying indicates the gold has absorbed into your skin. You will literally feel the skin tightening. It will feel good. Nothing else in this author's knowledge works so rapidly and effectively in combating wrinkles and bad skin. If its not working, then make sure its not past its expiration date. Also, with more purple flocculant in the bottle, the more high spin state gold has dropped out of its exotic matter status, and less gold is still in an ORMUS state. The purple particulate is colloidal gold, still beneficial, but not quite ORMUS. Once it starts turning dark purple it is not as bioavailable as when it is clear freshly made monatomic element.

# Gold with Light Therapy

A new field in modern therapeutic protocols is photo-medicine. It has been been shown that an appropriate dose of light can improve speed and quality of acute and chronic wound healing, soft tissue healing, and pain relief, improving immune system function and nerve regeneration.

Low-energy, non-ionizing, photon irradiation by light in the far-red and near-IR spectral range with low-energy (LLLT) lasers has been found to modulate various biological processes in cell cultures and in living organisms. This phenomenon of photobiomodulation has been applied clinically in the treatment of soft tissue injuries and shown acceleration of wound healing.

These types of light devices are sometimes referred to as Cold Lasers. Evidence suggests that cytochrome oxidase is a key photo acceptor of light in the far-red to near-IR spectral range. Cytochrome oxidase is an integral membrane protein that contains four redox active metal centers and has a strong absorbance in the far-red to near-IR spectral range increasing mitochondrial respiration and ATP synthesis in isolated mitochondria.

The mechanism of photobiomodulation by red to near-IR (infrared) light at the cellular level has been ascribed to the activation of mitochondrial electron transport chain components, resulting in initiation of a signaling cascade that promotes cellular proliferation and cytoprotection.

Science has recently discovered that low radiant exposure of near infrared light has profound effects on cellular functions. This includes improvement of wound healing; an increase of collagen production in human skin fibroblasts; an enhancement of oxidative metabolism in phagocytes; and proliferation of macrophages. In fact, it has recently been discovered that neurons themselves communicate in the 810nm wavelength.

Reduced gold (less than 5 nm), reflect this wavelength of near infrared, creating greater coherence and amplification of these cellular signals, thus explaining the improvement of cognitive abilities upon the therapeutic use of these gold compounds. In my own experiments I observed a doubling effect on collagen production. ORMUS Gold applied on the skin that was irradiated with a 810 nm Far-IR laser for 5-10 minutes showed twice the reduction in wrinkles. The other thing I noticed is repeated use is needed to keep the skin looking young and supple, yet with time the amount used can be decreased.

# Brain Health

It is this author's hypothesis that ORMUS Gold assists the growth of neural cells, especially ones in need of repair after damage. This is based on cross-correlating various scientific research that indicates that neurons communicate with each other using light signals in the infrared spectrum.

It turns out this wavelength of communication is precisely the wavelength reflected by nanoparticles of gold and thus the monatomic gold acts as a bio-amplifier and harmonizer for the neural signals, potentially causing the neurons to grow toward each other faster and in a more ordered fashion, even creating entirely new neural networks. This is called adult neurogenesis.

Nano preparations of gold have been proven in clinical trials to increase IQ, assist in recovery from addictions, alleviate depression, relieve anxiety and assist in treating other brain related issues improving mental balance, syncing the different parts of the brain together in harmony and coherence. My personal observations suggest nano gold, working as a catalyst, stimulates the growth of neurons, thereby repairing and rebuilding the neural pathways of the brain as well as increasing the overall conductivity of the synapses in the gray matter.

Perhaps the most astounding quality of gold is its effect on human intelligence. In a study at UCLA by Dr. Abrahams, subjects were found to have increased their IQ scores by 20% after taking colloidal gold for a short period of time!

Experiments were run on groups of people who were administered colloidal gold and placebo treatment; their IQs had been measured beforehand in order to detect the expected modifications.

The group who were administered nano gold for a month showed significant concentration capacity, whereas there was little modification in the case of those who were administered Placebo solutions. Nano gold administration was stopped for another month, and the study subjects were again tested; the IQ levels had remained superior to the before nano gold treatment figures. The test was repeated once more after two months with the same amazing effect. The encouraging results of many laboratory studies are the explanation for the increased use of nano gold in the treatment of the nervous disorders characterized by memory loss, lack of concentration and verbal deficiencies.

The cost of a colloidal gold treatment for IQ improvement is very low, which makes it possible for all social levels to benefit for it. Whether scholastically, educationally or medically used, it is an acknowledged fact already that nano gold increases IQ levels for an extended period of time. Reduced, high-spin, monatomic, nano, ORMUS or whatever you choose to call this gold, it has been used traditionally not only to improve the cognitive faculties of the brain, but to stabilize the emotional body and create aspirations for noble qualities. These include:

patience, peace, increased morale, positive attitude, attractive personality, intelligence, joy, happiness, emotional balance, calmness and equanimity. And let's not forget what may be the most important to many, a energetic libido and sex drive.

## Gold as Aphrodisiac

The joke goes that the number one aphrodisiac in the world is money, so gold, being the standard for all currencies on the planet is the best aphrodisiac we've got, both literally and figuratively. Gold has been found useful in cases of regulating and coordinating glandular and nervous systems because it helps to rejuvenate glands and stimulate nerves. It helps release pressure on neural pathways allowing nerve signals to function unimpeded and reach various organs and glands. My own observations are that the ingestion of ORMUS Gold is increased libido and sexual energy. Anything that increases cellular conductivity will do this. Greater vitality means greater procreative power.

Once I gave our ORMUS Gold to a couple in their early twenties and got an interesting testimonial back. This young man was complaining that his girlfriend, although very youthful and vibrant in appearance was suffering for more than two years from chronic fatigue, which was a source of frustration for both of them. I gave him a bottle of ORMUS.

I didn't know what it would do, but always have been interested in seeing how it effects people as the testimonials I've gotten over the years have been varied, sensational and amusing, such mundane benefits as relieving muscle strains to mitigating hangover from excessive alcohol consumption to more serious claims like shrinking tumors and and even esoteric reports of past life regression and not easily understood phenomenon of karmic cleansing, which is purely in the realm of either the supernatural, or a rich imagination.

But in this case, the man came back to me a few days later and said he gave his girlfriend three droppers of ORMUS Gold. The next day her chronic fatigue disappeared, and she became highly aroused and very passionate, keeping him in bed for two days. Needless to say he was a very happy man. I continued to send him bottles for a few years overseas. He wouldn't spare any expense to have it! We should all be so lucky. And in fact, one thing is certain, gold in its bioavailable state does something very beneficial to our bodies.

# Evidence of Gold's Therapeutic Use in the Bible

Secular science can say what it wants but sometimes the answer is right there in your own history. Some of the oldest known records of gold's use for human health is evidenced from passages within the Old Testament.

Exodus 32, Verse 19-20:

And it came to pass, as soon as he came nigh unto the camp, that he saw the calf, and the dancing: and Moses' anger waxed hot, and he cast the tables out of his hands, and brake them beneath the mount. And he took the golden calf which they had made, and burnt it in the fire, and ground it to powder, and strew it upon the water, and made the children of Israel drink of it.

Psalm 105: 37

He (Moses) brought them forth also with silver and gold: and there was not one feeble person among their tribes.

In fact, in Exodus, when Moses asked someone to make the "Bread of the Presence of God," who did he charge with this task?

It was Bazaleel, the blacksmith! Bazaleel's workshop for making this gold elixir was on the peak of Mt. Horeb. This is where they made the white powder of gold they called ShemManna and Mkfzt. Deciphered hieroglyphics in Egypt describe that this substance occupied space, had a physical mass, yet was so very weightless that "a feather could tip the scales against it". This is consistent with our own observations in making ORMUS Gold in our laboratory. The Exodus account of Moses melting down the golden calf and giving the subsequent gold elixir to his people can be said that this is the first written record in the history of mankind of gold being used therapeutically, in this case indicated for anxiety, impatience and downright stupidity.

## Conclusion + Bonus

If at this point one does not believe that gold in its reduced nano phase or what can be called its alchemical form does not have any health benefit, then no further convincing is possible. The overwhelming evidence of gold's therapeutic use from ancient to modern times is quite overwhelming, spanning everything from mainstream medicine to the mystical and esoteric.

I feel that I have benefited greatly in my health and mental balance and acuity from taking the ORMUS Gold made in our lab. To me, gold, properly reduced to its monatomic form and even as a colloidal, truly is the elixir of the ageless. As mentioned previously, much of my research and lab work was inspired by words written down many centuries ago. Standing on the shoulders of giants is both a humbling and empowering experience and there is still so much to be discovered from our antiquity that has been lost in the annals of history.

I'm including in this book two of my favorite alchemical texts. Fortunately, they are not covered by copyright, so I can share them herein. The first, the 'Tractatus Aureusi' or Golden Treatise of Hermes is one of the most complete and mysterious ancient writings on alchemy and has served as instruction and inspiration for many alchemists throughout the ages. Many years studying this cryptic text is no guarantee that its secrets will be revealed. The second is a translation of the 'Book of the Revelation of Hermes' as interpreted by Theophrastus Paracelsus and concerns the "Supreme Secret of the World." It was first published under the auspices of Benedictus Figulus in his 'Golden and Blessed Casket of Nature's Marvels,' in 1608.

## Bonus 1: 'Tractatus Aureus'

Even thus saith Hermes:

Through long years I have not ceased to experiment, neither have I spared any labour of mind, and this science and art I have obtained by the sole inspiration of the Living God, who judged fit to open them to me His servant, who has given to rational creatures the power of thinking and judging aright, forsaking none or giving to any occasion to despair.

For myself, I had never discovered this matter to anyone had it not been from fear of the judgment and the perdition of my soul, if I concealed it. It is a debt which I am desirous to discharge to the faithful as the Father of the faithful did liberally bestow it upon me. Understand ye then, O Sons of Wisdom, that the knowledge of the four elements of the ancient philosophers was not corporally or imprudently sought after, which are through patience to be discovered according to their causes and their occult operation. But, their operation is occult, since nothing is done except the matter be decompounded and because it is not perfected unless the colours be thoroughly passed and accomplished.

Know then, that the division that was made upon the water, by the ancient philosophers, separates it into four substances, one into two, and three into one, the third part of which is colour, as it were--a coagulated moisture; but the second and third waters are the Weights of the Wise. Take of the humidity, or moisture, an ounce and a half, and of the Southern Redness, which is the soul of gold, a fourth part, that is to say, half an ounce; of the citrine Seyre, in like manner, half an ounce; of the Auripigment, half an ounce, which are eight; that is three ounces. And know ye that the vine of the wise is drawn forth in three, but the wine thereof is not perfected, until at length thirty be accomplished. Understand the operation, therefore.

Decoction lessens the matter, but the tincture augments it, because Luna in fifteen days is diminished, and in the third she is augmented. This is the beginning and the end. Behold, I have declared that which was hidden, since the work is both with thee and about thee; that which was within is taken out and fixed, and thou canst have it either in earth or sea.

Keep, therefore, the Argent vive, which is prepared in the innermost chamber in which it is coagulated; for that is the Mercury which is celebrated from the residual earth. He, therefore, who now hears my words, let him search into them, which are to justify no evildoer, but to benefit the good; therefore I have discovered all things that were before hidden concerning this knowledge, and disclosed the greatest of all secrets, even the Intellectual Science. Know ye, therefore, Children of Wisdom, who inquire concerning the report thereof, that the vulture standing upon the mountain crieth out with a loud voice: 'I am the White of the Black, and the Red of the White, and the Citrine of the Red, and behold I speak the very Truth.' And know that the chief principle of the art is the Crow, which is the blackness of the night and the clearness of the day, and flies without wings.

From the bitterness existing in the throat the tincture is taken, the red goes forth from his body, and from his back is taken a thin water. Understand, therefore, and accept this gift of God which is hidden from the thoughtless world. In the caverns of the metals there is hidden the stone that is venerable, splendid in colour, a mind sublime and an open sea. Behold, I have declared it unto thee; give thanks to God who teacheth thee this knowledge, for He in return recompenses the grateful.

Put the matter into a moist fire, therefore, and cause it to boil, in order that its heat may be augmented, which destroys the siccity of the incombustible nature, until the radix shall appear; then extract the redness and the light parts, till only about a third remains. Sons of Science! For this reason are philosophers said to be envious, not that they grudged truth to religious or just men, or to the wise, but to fools, ignorant and vicious, who are without Self-Control and benevolence, lest they should be made powerful, and able to perpetrate sinful things.

For of such the philosophers are made accountable to God, and evil men are not admitted worthy of this wisdom. Know that this matter I call the stone, but it is also named the feminine of magnesia, or the hen, or the white spittle, or the volatile milk, the incombustible oil, in order that it may be hidden from the inept and ignorant, who are deficient in goodness and self-control; which I have nevertheless signified to the wise by one only epithet, viz., the Philosophers' Stone. Include, therefore, and conserve in this sea, the fire, and the heavenly bird, to the latest moment of his exit.

But I deprecate ye all, Sons of Philosophy, on whom the great gift of this knowledge being bestowed, if any should undervalue or divulge the power thereof to the ignorant, or such as are unfit for the knowledge of this secret. Behold, I have received nothing from any to whom I have not returned that which had been given me, nor have I failed to honour him; even in this I have reposed the highest confidence.

This, O Son, is the concealed Stone of many colours, which is born and brought forth in one colour; I know this and conceal it. By this, the Almighty favouring, the greatest diseases are escaped, and every sorrow, distress and evil and hurtful thing is made to depart; for it leads from darkness into light, from this desert wilderness to a secure habitation, and from poverty and straits to a free and ample fortune.

My son, before all things I admonish thee to fear God, in whom is the strength of thy undertaking, and the bond of whatsoever thou meditatest to unloose; whatsoever thou hearest, consider it rationally. For I hold thee not to be a fool. Lay hold, therefore, of my instructions and meditate upon them, and so let thy heart be fitted also to conceive, as if thou was thyself the author of that which I now teach. If thou appliest cold to any nature that is hot, it will not hurt it; in like manner, he who is rational shuts himself within from the threshold of ignorance, lest supinely he should be deceived.

Take the flying bird and drown it flying, and divide and separate it from its pollutions, which yet hold it in death; draw it forth and repel it from itself, that it may live and answer thee, not by flying away into the regions above but by truly forbearing to fly. For if thou shalt deliver it out of its prison, after this thou shalt govern it according to Reason, and according to the days that I shall teach thee: then will it become a companion unto thee, and by it thou wilt become to be an honoured lord. Extract from the ray its shadow, and from the light its obscurity, by which the clouds hang over it and keep away the light: by means of its construction, also, and fiery redness, it is burned.

Take, my Son, this redness, corrupted with water, which is as a live coal holding fire, which if thou shalt withdraw so often until the redness is made pure, then it will associate with thee, by whom it was cherished, and in whom it rests. Return, then, O my Son, the coal being extinct in life, upon the water for thirty days, as I shall note to thee, and henceforth thou art a crowned king, resting over the fountain, and drawing from thence Auripigment dry without moisture. And now I have made the heart of the hearers, hoping in thee, to rejoice, even in their eyes, beholding thee in anticipation of that which thou possessest. Observe, then, that the water was first in the air, then in the earth; restore thou it also to the superiors by its proper windings and not foolishly altering it; then to the former spirit, gathered in its redness, let it be carefully conjoined.

Know, my Son, that the fatness of our earth is sulphur, the auripigment sirety, and colcothar which are also sulphur, of which auripigments sulphur, and such like, some are more vile than others, in which there is a diversity, of which kind also is the fat of gluey matters, such as are hair, nails, hoofs, and sulphur itself, and of the brain, which too is auripigment, of the like kind also are the lions' and cats' claws, which is sirety the fat of white bodies, and the fat of the two oriental quicksilvers, which sulphurs are hunted and retained by the bodies. I say, moreover, that this sulphur doth tinge and fix, and is held by the conjunction of the tinctures; oils also tinge, but fly away, which in the body are contained, which is a conjunction of fugitives only with sulphurs and albuminous bodies, which hold also and detain the fugitive ens.

The disposition sought after by the philosophers, O Son, is but one in our egg, but this in the hen's egg is much less to be found. But lest so much of the Divine Wisdom as is a hen's egg should not be distinguished, our composition is, as that is, from the four elements adapted and composed. Know, therefore, that in the hen's egg is the greatest help with respect to the proximity and relationship of the matter in nature for in it there is a spirituality and conjunction of elements, and an earth which is golden in its tincture.

But the Son, inquiring of Hermes, saith:

The sulphurs which are fit for our work, whether they are celestial or terrestrial?

To whom the Father replies:

Certain of them are heavenly and some are of the earth.

Then the Son saith:

Father, I imagine the heart in the superiors to be heaven, and in the inferiors, earth.

But saith Hermes:

It is not so; the masculine is truly the heaven of the feminine, and the feminine is the earth of the masculine.

The Son then asks:

Father, which of these is more worthy than the other, whether is it the heaven or the earth?

Hermes replies:

Both need the help one of the other, for the precepts demand a medium.

But saith the Son:

If thou shalt say that a wise man governs all mankind?

But ordinary men, replies Hermes, are better for them, because every nature delights in society of its own kind, and so we find it to be in the life of Wisdom where equals are conjoined.

But what," rejoins the Son, "is the mean betwixt them?

To whom Hermes replies:

In everything in nature there are three from two; the beginning, the middle, and the end. First the needful water, then the oily tincture, and lastly, the faeces, or earth, which remains below. But the Dragon inhabits in all these, and his houses are the darkness and blackness that is in them, and by them he ascends into the air, from his rising, which is their heaven. But whilst the fume remains in them, they are not immortal. Take away, therefore, the vapour from the water, and the blackness from the oily tincture, and death from the faeces, and by dissolution thou shalt possess a triumphant reward, even that in and by which the possessors live.

Know then, my Son, that the temperate unguent, which is fire, is the medium between the faeces and the water, and is the Perscrutinator of the water. For the unguents are called sulphurs, because between fire and oil and this sulphur there is such a close proximity, that even as fire burns so does the sulphur also. All the sciences of the world, O Son, are comprehended in this my hidden Wisdom, and this, and the learning of the Art, consists in these wonderful hidden elements which it doth discover and complete.

It behoves him, therefore, who would be introduced to this hidden Wisdom, to free himself from the hidden usurpations of vice, and to be just and good and of a sound reason, ready at hand to help mankind, of a serene countenance, diligent to save, and be himself a patient guardian of the arcane secrets of philosophy. And this know, that except thou understandest how to mortify and induce generation, to vivify the Spirit and introduce Light, until they fight each other and grow white and freed from their defilements, rising as it were from blackness and darkness, thou knowest nothing nor canst perform anything. But if thou knowest this, thou wilt be of a great dignity so that even kings themselves shall reverence thee.

These secrets, Son, it behoves thee to conceal from the vulgar and profane world. Understand, also, that our Stone is from many things and of various colours, and composed from four elements which we ought to divide and dissever in pieces, and segregate, in the veins, and partly mortifying the same by its proper nature, which is also in it, to preserve the water and fire dwelling therein, which is from the four elements and their waters, which contain its water; this, however, is not water in its true form, but fire, containing in a pure vessel the ascending waters, lest the spirits should fly away from the bodies; for by this means they are made tingeing and fixed.

O, blessed watery form, that dissolvest the elements! Now it behoves us, with this watery soul, to possess ourselves of a sulphurous form, and to mingle the same with our Acetum. For when, by the power of water, the composition is dissolved, it is the key of the restoration; then darkness and death will fly away from them and Wisdom proceeds onwards to the fulfilment of her Law.

Know, my Son, that the philosophers bind up their matter with a strong chain that it may contend with the Fire; because the spirits in the washed bodies desire to dwell therein and to rejoice. In these habitations they vivify themselves and inhabit there, and the bodies hold them, nor can they be hereafter separated any more. The dead elements are revived, the composed bodies tinge and are altered, and by a wonderful process they are made permanent, as saith the philosopher.

O, permanent watery Form, creatrix of the royal elements! who, having with thy brethren and a just government obtained the tincture, findest rest. Our precious stone is cast forth upon the dung-hill, and that which is most worthy is made vilest of the vile. Therefore, it behoves us to mortify two Argent vives together, both to venerate and be venerated, viz., the Argent vive of Auripigment, and the oriental Argent vive of Magnesia. O, Nature, the most potent creatrix of Nature, which containest and separatist natures in a middle principle.

The Stone comes with light, and with light it is generated, and then it generates and brings forth the black clouds of darkness, which is the mother of all things. But when we marry the crowned King to our red daughter, and in a gentle fire, not hurtful she doth

Conceive an excellent and supernatural son, which permanent life she doth also feed with a subtle heat, so that he lives at length in our fire.

But when thou shalt send forth thy fire upon the foliated sulphur, the boundary of hearts doth enter in above, it is washed in the same, and the purified matter thereof is extracted. Then he is transformed, and his tincture by help of the fire remains red, as it were flesh. But our Son, the king begotten, takes his tincture from the fire, and death even, and darkness, and the waters flee away.

The Dragon shuns the sunbeams which dart through the crevices and our dead son lives; the king comes forth from the fire and rejoins with his spouse, the occult treasures are laid open, and the virgin's milk is whitened. The Son, already vivified, is become a warrior in the fire, and of tincture super-excellent. For this Son is himself the treasury, even himself bearing the Philosophic Matter. Approach, ye Sons of wisdom, and rejoice; let us now rejoice together, for the reign of death is finished, and the Son doth rule. And he is invested with the red garment, and the scarlet colour is put on.

Understand, then, O Son of Wisdom, what the Stone declares: 'Protect me and I will protect Thee; increase my strength that I may help thee! My Sol and my beams are most inward and secretly in me, my own Luna, also, is my light, exceeding every other light, and my good things are better than all other good things, I give freely, and reward the intelligent with joy and gladness, glory, riches, and delights, and them that seek after me I make to know and understand, and to possess divine things.'

Behold, that which the philosophers have concealed is written with seven letters; for Alpha and Yda follow two, and Sol in like manner follows the book. Nevertheless, if thou art willing that he should have Dominion, observe the Art, and join the son to the daughter of the water, which is Jupiter and a hidden secret. Auditor, understand. Let us use our Reason.

Consider all with the most accurate investigation, which in the contemplative part I have demonstrated to thee, the whole matter I know to be the one only thing. But who is he that understands the true investigation and inquires rationally into this matter? It is not from man, nor from anything like him or akin to him; nor from the ox or bullock, and if any creature conjoins with one of another species, that which is brought forth is neutral from either.

Thus saith Venus: 'I beget light, nor is the darkness of my nature, and if my metal be not dried all bodies desire me, for I liquefy them and wipe away their rust, even I extract their substance. Nothing, therefore is better or more venerable than I, my brother also being conjoined.' But the King, the Ruler, to his brethren, testifying of him, saith: 'I am crowned, and I am adorned with a royal diadem. I am clothed with the royal garment, and I bring joy and gladness of heart, for being chained, I caused my substance to lay hold of, and to rest within the arms and breast of my mother, and to fasten upon her substance, making that which was invisible to become visible, and the occult matter to appear. And everything which the philosophers have hidden is generated by us. Hear, then, these words, and understand them.

Keep them, and meditate thereon, and seek for nothing more. Man in the beginning is generated of nature, whose inward substance is fleshy, and not from anything else. Meditate on these plain things, and reject what is superfluous.'

Thus saith the philosopher: 'Botri is made from the citrine, which is extracted out of the Red Root, and from nothing else; and if it be citrine and nothing else Wisdom was with thee. It was not gotten by thy care, nor if it be freed from redness, by thy study. Behold, I have circumscribed nothing. If thou hast understanding, there be but few things unopened. Ye Sons of Wisdom! Turn then the Breym Body with an exceeding great fire, and it will yield gratefully what you desire. And see that you make that which is volatile, so that it cannot fly, and by means of that which flies not. And that which yet rests upon the fire, as it were itself a fiery flame, and that which in the heat of a boiling fire is corrupted, is cambar. And know ye that the Art of this permanent water is our brass and the colouring of its tincture and blackness is then changed into the true red.

I declare that, by the help of God, I have spoken nothing but the truth. That which is destroyed is renovated, and hence the corruption is made manifest in the matter to be renewed, and hence the melioration will appear, and on either side it is a signal of Art. My Son, that which is born of the Crow is the beginning of this Art.

Behold, now I have obscured the matter treated of, by circumlocution, depriving thee of the light. Yet this dissolved, this joined, this nearest and farthest off, I have named to thee. Roast those things, therefore, and boil them in that which comes from the horse's belly for seven, fourteen or twenty-one days. Then will the Dragon eat his own wings and destroy himself.

This being done, let it be put into a fiery furnace, which lute diligently, and observe that none of the spirit may escape. And know that the periods of the earth are in the water, which let it be as long as until thou puttest the same upon it. This matter being thus melted and burned, take the brain thereof and triturate it in most sharp vinegar, till it becomes obscured.

This done, it lives in the putrefaction, let the dark clouds which were in it before it was killed be converted into its own body. Let this process be repeated, as I have described, let it again die, as I before said, and then it lives. In the life and death thereof we work with the spirits, for as it dies by the taking away of the spirit, so it lives in the return and is revived and rejoices therein. Being arrived then at this knowledge, that which thou hast been searching for is made apparent in the Affirmation.

I have even related to thee the joyful signs, even that which doth fix the body. But these things, and how they attained to the knowledge of this secret, are given by our ancestors in figures and types. Behold, they are dead. I have opened the riddle, and the book of knowledge is revealed.

The hidden things I have uncovered, and have brought together the scattered truths within their boundary, and have conjoined many various forms; even I have associated the spirit. Take it as the gift of God. It behoves thee to give thanks to God, Who has bestowed liberally of his bounty to the Wise, Who delivers us from misery and poverty. I am tempted and proven with the fullness of His substance and His probable wonders, and humbly pray God that whilst we live we may come to Him.

Remove thence, O Sons of Science, the unguents which we extract from fats, hair, verdigrease, tragacanth and bones, which are written in the books of our fathers. But concerning the ointments which contain the tincture, coagulate the fugitive, and adorn the sulphurs, it behoves us to explain their disposition more at large, and to unveil the Form, which is buried and hidden from other unguents, which is seen in disposition, but dwells in his own body, as fire in trees and stones, which by the most subtle art and ingenuity it behoves to extract without burning. And know that the heaven is to be joined mediately with the earth, but the Form is in a middle nature between the heaven and the earth, which is our water.

But the water holds of all the first place which goes forth from this stone. But the second is gold, and the third is gold, only in a mean which is more noble than the water and the faeces. But in these are the smoke, the blackness and the death. It behoves us, therefore, to dry away the vapour from the water, to expel the blackness from the unguent, and death from the faeces and this by dissolution.

By which means we attain to the highest philosophy and secret of all hidden things. Know ye then, O Sons of Science, there are seven bodies, of which gold is the first, the most perfect, the king of them, and their head, which neither the earth can corrupt nor fire devastate, nor the water change for its complexion is equalized, and its nature regulated with respect to heat, cold and moisture; nor is there anything in it which is superfluous, therefore the philosophers do buoy up and magnify themselves in it, saying that this gold, in relation to other bodies is, as the sun amongst the stars, more splendid in Light; and as, by the power of God, every vegetable and all the fruits of the earth are perfected, so gold by the same power sustaineth all.

For as dough without a ferment cannot be fermented so when thou sublimest the body and purifiest it, separating the uncleanness from it, thou wilt then conjoin and mix them together, and put in the ferment confecting the earth and water. Then will the Ixir ferment even as dough doth ferment. Think of this, and see how the ferment in this case doth change the former nature's to another thing.

Observe also, that there is no ferment otherwise than from the dough itself. Observe, moreover, that the ferment whitens the confection and hinders it from turning, and holds the tincture lest it should fly, and rejoice the bodies, and makes them intimately to join and to enter one into another, and this is the key of the philosophers and the end of their work, and by this science, bodies are ameliorated, and the operation of them, God assisting, is consummate.

But, through negligence and a false opinion of the matter, the operation may be perverted, as a mass of leaven growing corrupt, or milk turned with rennet for cheese, and musk among aromatics. The sure colour of the golden matter for the red, and the nature thereof, is not sweetness; therefore we make of them sericum--i.e., Ixir; and of them we make the enamel of which we have already written, and with the king's seal we have tinged the clay, and in that have set the colour of heaven, which augments the sight of them that see. The Stone, therefore, is the most precious gold without spots, evenly tempered, which neither fire, nor air, nor water, nor earth is able to corrupt; for it is the Universal Ferment rectifying all things in a medium composition, whose complexion is yellow and a true citrine colour.

The gold of the wise, boiled and well digested, with a fiery water, makes Ixir, for the gold of the wise is more heavy than lead, which in a temperate composition is a ferment Ixir, and contrariwise, in our intemperate composition, is the confusion of the whole. For the work begins from the vegetable, next from the animal, as in a hen's egg, in which is the greatest help, and our earth is gold, all of which we make sericum, which is the ferment Ixir.

# BONUS 2: THE BOOK OF THE REVELATION OF HERMES

*As Interpreted by Theophrastus Paracelsus Concerning The Supreme Secret of the World.'*

Hermes, Plato, Aristotle, and the other philosophers, flourishing at different times, who have introduced the Arts, and more especially have explored the secrets of inferior creation, all these have eagerly sought a means whereby man's body might be preserved from decay and become endued with immortality.

To them it was answered that there is nothing which might deliver the mortal body from death; but that there is One Thing which may postpone decay, renew youth, and prolong short human life (as with the Patriarchs).

For death was laid as a punishment upon our first parents, Adam and Eve, and will never depart from all their descendants. Therefore, the above philosophers, and many others, have sought this One Thing with great labour, and have found that which preserves the human body from corruption, and prolongs life, conducts itself, with respect to other elements, as it were like the Heavens from which they understood that the Heavens are a substance above the Four Elements. And just as the Heavens, with respect to the other elements are held to be the fifth substance (for they are indestructible, stable, and suffer no foreign admixture), so also this One Thing (compared to the forces of our body) is an indestructible essence, drying up all the superfluities of our bodies, and has been philosophically called by the above-mentioned name.

It is neither hot and dry like fire, nor cold and moist like water, nor warm and moist like air, nor dry and cold like earth. But it is a skilful, perfect equation of all the Elements, a right commingling of natural forces, a most particular union of spiritual virtues, an indissoluble uniting of body and soul. It is the purest and noblest substance of an indestructible body, which cannot be destroyed nor harmed by the Elements, and is produced by Art.

With this Aristotle prepared an apple prolonging life by its scent, when he, fifteen days before his death, could neither eat nor drink on account of old age. This spiritual Essence, or One Thing, was revealed from above to Adam, and was greatly desired by the Holy Fathers, this also Hermes and Aristotle call the Truth without Lies, the most sure of all things certain, the Secret of all Secrets.

It is the Last and the Highest Thing to be sought under the Heavens, a wondrous closing and finish of philosophical work, by which are discovered the dews of Heaven and the fastnesses of Earth. What the mouth of man cannot utter is all found in this Spirit. As Morienus says: 'He who has this has all things, and wants no other aid. For in it are all temporal happiness, bodily health, and earthly fortune. It is the spirit of the fifth substance, a Fount of all Joys (beneath the rays of the moon), the Supporter of Heaven and Earth, the Mover of Sea and Wind, the Outpourer of Rain, upholding the strength of all things, an excellent spirit above Heavenly and other spirits, giving Health, Joy, Peace, Love: driving away Hatred and Sorrow, bringing in Joy, expelling all Evil, quickly healing all Diseases, destroying Poverty and Misery, leading to all good things, preventing all evil words and thoughts, giving man his heart's desire, bringing to the pious earthly honour and long life, but to the wicked who misuse it, Eternal Punishment.'

This is the Spirit of Truth, which the world cannot comprehend without the interposition of the Holy Ghost, or without the instruction of those who know it. The same is of a mysterious nature, wondrous strength, boundless power. The Saints, from the beginning of the world, have desired to behold its face. By Avicenna this Spirit is named the Soul of the World.

For as the Soul moves all the limbs of the Body, so also does this Spirit move all bodies. And as the Soul is in all the limbs of the Body, so also is this Spirit in all elementary created things. It is sought by many and found by few. It is beheld from afar and found near; for it exists in every thing, in every place, and at all times. It has the powers of all creatures; its action is found in all elements, and the qualities of all things are therein, even in the highest perfection. By virtue of this essence did Adam and the Patriarchs preserve their health and live to an extreme age, some of them also flourishing in great riches.

When the philosophers had discovered it, with great diligence and labour, they straightway concealed it under a strange tongue, and in parables, lest the same should become known to the unworthy, and the pearls be cast before swine. For if everyone knew it, all work and industry would cease; man would desire nothing but this one thing, people would live wickedly, and the world be ruined, seeing that they would provoke God by reason of their avarice and superfluity.

For eye hath not seen, nor ear heard, nor hath the heart of man understood what Heaven hath naturally incorporated with this Spirit. Therefore have I briefly enumerated some of the qualities of this Spirit, to the Honour of God, that the pious may reverently praise Him in His gifts (which gift of God shall afterwards come to them), and I will herewith shew what powers and virtues it possesses in each thing, also its outward appearance, that it may be more readily recognized.

In its first state, it appears as an impure earthly body, full of imperfections. It then has an earthly nature, healing all sickness and wounds in the bowels of man, producing good and consuming proud flesh, expelling all stench, and healing generally, inwardly and outwardly. In its second nature, it appears as a watery body, somewhat more beautiful than before, because (although still having its corruptions) its Virtue is greater. It is much nearer the Truth, and more effective in works. In this form it cures cold and hot fevers, and is a specific against poisons, which it drives from heart and lungs, healing the same when injured or wounded, purifying the blood, and, taken three times a day, is of great comfort in all diseases.

But in its third nature it appears as an aerial body of an oily nature, almost freed from all imperfections, in which form it does many wondrous works, producing beauty and strength of body, and (a small quantity being taken in the food) preventing melancholy and heating of the gall, increasing the quantity of blood and seed. It expands the blood vessels, cures withered limbs, restores strength to the sight, in growing persons removes what is superfluous and makes good defects in the limbs.

In its fourth nature it appears in a fiery form (not quite freed from all imperfections, still somewhat watery and not dried enough), wherein it has many virtues making the old young and reviving those at the point of death. For if to such an one there be given, in wine, a barleycorn's weight of this fire, so that it reach the stomach, it goes to his heart, renewing him at once, driving away all previous moisture and poison, and restoring the natural heat of the liver.

Given in small doses to old people, it removes the diseases of age, giving the old young hearts and bodies. Hence it is called the Elixir of Life. In its fifth and last nature, it appears in a glorified and illuminated form, without defects, shining like gold and silver, wherein it possesses all previous powers and virtues in a higher and more wondrous degree. Here its natural works are taken for miracles. When applied to the roots of dead trees they revive, bringing forth leaves and fruit.

A lamp, the oil of which is mingled with this spirit, continues to burn for ever without diminution. It converts crystals into the most precious stones of all colours, equal to those from the mines, and does many other incredible wonders which may not be revealed to the unworthy.

For it heals all dead and living bodies without other medicine. Here Christ is my witness that I lie not, for all heavenly influences are united and combined therein. This essence also reveals all treasures in earth and sea, converts all metallic bodies into gold, and there is nothing like unto it under Heaven.

This spirit is the secret, hidden from the beginning yet granted by God to a few holy men for the revealing of these riches to His Glory dwelling in fiery form in the air, and leading earth with itself to Heaven, while from its body there flow whole rivers of living water.

This spirit flies through the midst of the Heavens like a morning mist, leads its burning fire into the water, and has its shining realm in the Heavens. And although these writings may be regarded as false by the reader, yet to the initiated they are true and possible, when the hidden sense is properly understood. For God is wonderful in His works, and His wisdom is without end.

This spirit in its fiery form is called a Sandaraca, in the aerial a Kybrick, in the watery an Azoth, in the earthly Alcohoph and Aliocosoph. Hence they are deceived by these names, who, seeking without instruction, think to find this Spirit of Life in things foreign to our Art.

For although this Spirit which we seek, on account of its qualities, is called by these names, yet the same is not in these bodies and cannot be in them. For a refined spirit cannot appear except in a body suitable to its nature. And, by however many names it be called, let no one imagine there be different spirits, for, say what one will, there is but one spirit working everywhere and in all things.

That is the spirit which, when rising, illumines the Heavens, when setting incorporates the purity of Earth, and when brooding has embraced the Waters. This spirit is named Raphael, the Angel of God, the subtlest. and purest, whom the others all obey as their King.

This spiritual substance is neither heavenly nor hellish, but an airy, pure, and hearty body, midway between the highest and the lowest, without reason, but fruitful in works, and the most select and beautiful of all other heavenly things.

This work of God is far too deep for understanding for it is the last, greatest, and highest secret of Nature. It is the Spirit of God, which in the Beginning filled the Earth and brooded over the waters, which the world cannot grasp without the gracious interposition of the Holy Spirit and instruction from those who know it, which also the whole world desires for its virtue, and which cannot be prized enough.

For it reaches to the planets, raises the clouds, drives away mists, gives its light to all things, turns everything into Sun and Moon, bestows all health and abundance of treasure, cleanses the leper, brightens the eyes, banishes sorrow, heals the sick, reveals all hidden treasures, and, generally, cures all diseases.

Through this spirit have the philosophers invented the Seven Liberal Arts, and thereby gained their riches. Through the same Moses made the golden vessels in the Ark, and King Solomon did many beautiful works to the honour of God. Therewith Moses built the Tabernacle, Noah the Ark, Solomon the Temple. By this Ezra restored the Law, and Miriam, Moses' sister, was hospitable; Abraham, Isaac, and Jacob, and other righteous men, have had life-long abundance and riches; and all the saints possessing it have therewith praised God.

Therefore is its acquisition very hard, more than that of gold and silver. For it is the best of all things, because, of all things mortal that man can desire in this world, nothing can compare with it, and in it alone is truth. Hence it is called the Stone and Spirit of Truth; in its works is no vanity, its praise cannot be sufficiently expressed. I am unable to speak enough of its virtues, because it's good qualities and powers are beyond human thoughts, unutterable by the tongue of man, and in it are found the properties of all things.

Yea, there is nothing deeper in Nature. O unfathomable abyss of God's Wisdom, which thus hath united and comprised in the virtue and power of this one Spirit the qualities of all existing bodies! O unspeakable honour and boundless joy granted to mortal man! For the destructible things of Nature are restored by virtue of the said Spirit. O mystery of mysteries, most secret of all secret things, and healing and medicine of all things!

Thou last discovery in earthly natures, last best gift to Patriarchs and Sages, greatly desired by the Whole world! Oh, what a wondrous and laudable spirit is purity, in which stand all joy, riches, fruitfulness of life, and art of all arts, a power which to its initiates grants all material joys!

O desirable knowledge, lovely above all things beneath the circle of the Moon, by which Nature is strengthened, and heart and limbs are renewed, blooming youth is preserved, old age driven away, weakness destroyed, beauty in its perfection preserved, and abundance ensured in all things pleasing to men! O thou spiritual substance, lovely above all things! O thou wondrous power, strengthening all the world! O thou invincible virtue, highest of all that is, although despised by the ignorant, yet held by the wise in great praise, honour, and glory, that-- proceeding from humours--wakest the dead, expellest diseases, restorest the voice of the dying! 0 thou treasure of treasures, mystery of mysteries, called by Avicenna 'an unspeakable substance,' the purest and most perfect soul of the world, than which there is nothing more costly under Heaven, unfathomable in nature and power, wonderful in virtue and works, having no equal among creatures, possessing the virtues of all bodies under Heaven!

For from it flow the water of life, the oil and honey of eternal healing, and thus hath it nourished them with honey and water from the rock. Therefore, saith Morienus: 'He who hath it, the same also hath all things.' Blessed art Thou, Lord God of our Fathers, in that Thou has given the prophets this knowledge and understanding, that they have hidden these things (lest they should be discovered by the blind, and those drowned in worldly godlessness) by which the wise and pious have praised Thee!

For the discoverers of the mystery of this Thing to the unworthy are breakers of the seal of Heavenly Revelation, thereby offending God's Majesty, and bringing upon themselves many misfortunes and the punishments of God. Therefore, I beg all Christians, possessing this knowledge, to communicate the same to nobody, except it be to one living in Godliness, of well-proved virtue, and praising God, Who has given such a treasure to man.

For many seek, but few find it. Hence the impure and those living in vice are unworthy of it. Therefore is this Art to be shown to all God-fearing persons, because it cannot be bought with a price. I testify before God that I lie not, although it appear impossible to fools, that no one has hitherto explored Nature so deeply.

The Almighty be praised for having created this Art and for revealing it to God-fearing men. And thus is fulfilled this precious and excellent work, called the revealing of the occult spirit, in which lie hidden the secrets and mysteries of the world. But this spirit is one genius, and Divine, wonderful and lordly power. For it embraces the whole world, and overcomes the Elements and the fifth Substance.

*To our Trismegistus Spagyrus, Jesus Christ, Be praise and glory immortal. At one.*

# BIBLIOGRAPHY

1) Petrucci F, et al. "Biomonitoring of a worker population exposed to platinum dust in a catalyst production plant." Occupational and Environmental Medicine, 2005; 62:27-33.

2) Melichar B, et al. "Gastrointestinal permeability in ovarian cancer and breast cancer patients treated with Paclitaxel and platinum." BMC Cancer, 2007; 7:155.

3) Hainfeld JF. "A small gold-conjugated antibody label: Improved resolution for electron microscopy." Science, 1987;236:450.

4) Frens G. "Controlled nucleation for the regulation of the particle size in monodisperse gold suspensions." Nature Phy Sci, 1973; 241:20-22.

5) Horisberger M and Rosset J. "Colloidal gold: A useful marker for transmission and scanning electron microscopy." J Histochem & Cytochem, 1977; 25:295-305.

6) Goodman SL, Hodges GM, et al. "A review of the colloidal gold marker system." Scan Electron Microscopy, 1980; 11:133- 146.

7) Everett DH. Basic Principles of Colloid Science. The Royal Society of Chemistry, London, 1988; 5-36.

8) De Roe C, Courtoy PJ, et al. "A model of protein-colloidal gold interactions." J Histochem & Cytochem, 1987; 35:1191-1198.

9) Sutton BM and Dimartino M. "Gold." In: Handbook on Toxicity of Inorganic Compounds. Seiler HG and Sigel H, editors. Marcel Dekker, Inc., New York, 1988; 307-314.

10) Goodman & Gilman's: The Pharmacological Basis of Therapeutics. McGraw-Hill, New York, 1996; 644-646.

11) Mahdihassan S. "Cinnabar-gold as the best alchemical drug of longevity, called makaradhwaja in India." Am J Chinese Med, 1985; 13:93-108.

12) "Exodus (32:19-20)." The Oxford Study Bible. Oxford University Press, New York, 1992.

13) Higby GJ. "Gold in medicine, A review of its use in the West before 1900." Gold Bulletin, 1982; 15:130-140.

14) Weiser HB. Inorganic Colloidal Gold Chemistry. Wiley, New York, 1933; 1:21-57.

15) Faraday MX. "The Bakerian Lecture — Experimental relations of gold (and other metals) to light." Phil Trans R Soc Lond, 1857; 147:145-181.

16) Horisberger M. "The gold method as applied to lectin cytochemistry in transmission and scanning electron microscopy." Technique in Immunocytochemistry, 1985; 3:155-178.

17) Glazman YM. "Effect of surface-active agents on stability of hydrophobic sols." Faraday Discuss, 1966; 42:255-266.

18) Hawkins HK, Rehm LZ, et al. "Colloidal gold labeling of sections and cell surfaces." Ultrastructural Pathol, 1992; 16:61- 70.

19) Maclagan NF. "The preparation and use of colloidal gold sols as diagnostic agents." J Exp Path, 1947; 27: 369-377.

20) Komiyama A and Spicer SS. "Microendocytosis in eosinophillic leukocytes." J Cell Biol, 1975; 64:622-635.

21) Aonuma K. "Colloidal gold uptake as a marker for monocyte differentiation and maturation in normal and leukemic cells." Int'l Hematology, 1992; 55:265-274.

22) Feldherr C and Akin D. "The permeability of nuclear envelope in dividing and nondividing cell culture." J Cell Biol, 1990; 111:1-8.

23) Feldherr C and Akin D. "Signal-mediated nuclear transport in proliferating and growth-arrested BALA/c 3T3 cells." J Cell Biol, 1991; 115:933-939.

24) Danien BJ, Sims PA, et al. "Use of colloidal gold and neutron activation in correlative microscopic labeling and label quantitation." Scanning Microscopy, 1995; 9:773-780.

25) Ackerman GAM and Wolken KW. "Histochemical evidence for the differential surface labeling. Uptake, and intracellular transport of a colloidal gold-labeled insulin complex by normal human blood cells." J Histochem & Cytochem, 1981; 29:1137- 1149.

26) De Roe C, Courtoy PJ, et al. "Molecular aspects of the interactions between protein, colloidal gold and cultured cells: Applications to galactosylated serum albumin and rat hepatocytes." Arch Intern Physiol Biochem, 1982; 90:186.

27) Juurlink BHJ and Devon RM. "Colloidal gold as a permanent marker of cells." Experientia, 1991; 47:75-77.

28) Garner M, Rglinski J, et al. "The interaction of colloidal metal with erythrocytes." J Inorg Biochem, 1994; 56:283-290.

29) Lazareic MB, Yan K, et al. "Effect of gold compounds on the activity of adenylyl cyclase in human lymphocyte membranes." Arthritis & Rheumatism, 1992; 35:857-864.

30) Vint IAM, Foreman JC, et al. "The gold antirheumatic drug Auranofin governs T-cell activation by

enhancing oxygen free radical production." Eur J Immunol, 1994; 24:1961-1965.

31) Sato H, Yamaguvhi M, et al. "Induction of stress proteins in mouse peritoneal macrophages by the anti-rheumatic agents gold sodium thiomalate and Auranofin." Biochem Pharmacol, 1995; 49:1453-1457.

32) Cahill RNP. "Effect of sodium aurothiomalate myocrisin on DNA synthesis in phytohaemagglutin-stimulated cultures of sheep lymphocytes." Experientia, 1971; 27:913-914.

33) Lorbat A, Simon T, et al. "Chrysotherapy, suppression of immunoglobulin synthesis." Arthritis Rheum, 1978; 21:785- 791.

34) Forestier J. "La chrysotherapie dans les rhumatismes chroniques." Bull et Mem Soc Med des Hop de Paris, 1929; 44:323-329.

35) Forestier J. "Rheumatoid arthritis and its treatment by gold salts." J Lab Clin Med, 1935; 20:827-840.

36) Empire Rheumatism Council. "Gold therapy in rheumatoid arthritis. Final report of a multicenter controlled trial." Ann Rheum Dis, 1961; 20:315-324.

37) Geddes DM and Brostoff J. "Pulmonary fibrosis associated with hypersensitivity to gold salts." BMJ, 1976; 1:1444.

38) Gould PW, McCormack PL, et al. "Pulmonary damage associated with sodium aurothiomalate therapy." J Rheumatol, 1977; 3:181-182.

39) Scott DL, Bradby GV, et al. "Relationship of gold and penicillamine therapy to diffuse intestinal lung disease." Ann Rheum Dis, 1981; 40:136-141.

40) Belleli A, Boiardi L, et al. "Diffuse intestinal lung disease associated with hypersensitivity to gold salt." Clin Exp Rheumatol, 1985; 3:181-182.

41) Kay AGL. "Myelotoxicity of gold." BMJ, 1976; I:1266-1268.

42) Coblyn JS, Weinblatt M, et al. "Gold-induced thrombocytopaenia; A clinical and immunogenetic study of twenty-three patients." Ann Intern Med, 1981; 95:178-181.

43) Adachi JD, Benson WG, et al. "Gold-induced thrombocytopaenia; 12 Cases and a review of the literature." Semin Arthritis Rheum, 1987; 16:287-293.

44) Amos RS and Bax DE. "Leucopaenia in rheumatoid arthritis: Relationship to gold or sulphasalazine therapy." Br J Rheum, 1988; 27:465-468.

45) Madhok R, Pullar T, et al. "Chrysotherapy and thrombocytopenia." Ann Rheum Dis, 1985; 44:589-591.

46) Epstein WV, Henke CJ, et al. "Effect of parenterally administered gold therapy on the course of adult rheumatoid arthritis." Ann Int Med, 1991; 114:437-444.

47) Finkelstein AE, Walz DT, et al. "Auranofin: New oral gold compound for treatment of rheumatoid arthritis." Ann Rheum Dis, 1976; 35:251-257.

48) Pearson RG. "Hard and soft acids and bases." J of Amer Chemical Society, 1963; 85:3533-3539.

49) Kligman AM. "The identification of contact allergens by human assay. III. The Maximization Test: A procedure for screening and rating contact sensitizers." J Invest Derm, 1966; 47:393-409.

50) Hardcastle J, Hardcastle PT, et al. "Effect of Auranofin on ion transport by rat small intestine." J Pharm Pharmacol, 1989;41:817-823.

51) Lockie LM and Smith DM. "Forty-seven years experience with gold therapy in 1019 rheumatoid arthritis patients." Semin Arthritis Rheum, 1985; 14:238-246.

52) Panayi GS. "New ideas on the pathogenesis of rheumatoid arthritis." Ann Ital Med Int, 1990; 5:1-4.

53) Abraham GE and Himmel PB. "Management of rheumatoid arthritis: Rationale for the use of colloidal

metallic gold." Journal of Nut and Env Med, 1997; 7:295-305.

54) Pincus T, Summey JA, et al. "Assessment of patient satisfaction in activities of daily living using a modified Stanford Health Assessment Questionnaire." Arthritis Rheum, 1983; 26:1346- 1353.

55) Lansbury J. "Quantitation of the activity of rheumatoid arthritis." Am J Med Sci, 1956; 232:300-310.

56) American Rheumatology Association. Dictionary of Rheumatic Diseases, Vol. I. Signs and Symptoms. Contact Associates International Ltd, New York, 1992.

57) Abraham GE, McReynolds SA, et al. "Effects of colloidal metallic gold on cognitive functions: A pilot study." Frontier Perspective, 1998; 7:39-41.

58) Lezak MD. Neuropsychological Assessment. Oxford University Press, New York, 1995; 690.

59) Lezak MD. Neuropsychological Assessment. Oxford University Press, New York, 1995; 691.

60) McDowell I and Newell C. Measuring Health — A Guide to Rating Scales and Questionnaires. Oxford University Press, Inc, New York, 1987; 249-252.

61) Belza BL. "Comparison of self-reported fatigue in rheumatoid arthritis and controls." Journal of Rheumatology, 1995; 22:639-643.

62) DeJong RN. The Neurologic Examination. Harper and Row, New York, 1967; 524-559.

63) Benedict R and Horton AM. "The construct validity of the fourword short-term memory test: A preliminary study." International Journal of Neuroscience, 1990; 2:199-202.

64) Chevallet M, Luche S, et al. "Silver staining of proteins in polyacrylamide gels." National Protoc, 2006; 1:1852-1858.

65) Uchihara T. "Silver diagnosis in neuropathology: Principles, practice, and revised interpretation." Acta Neuropathoi (Berl), 2007; 113:483-499.

66) Babu R, Zhang J, et al. "Antimicrobial activities of silver used as a polymerization catalyst for wound-healing matrix." Biomaterials, 2006; 27:4304-4313.

67) Feng OL, Wu J, et al. "A Mechanistic study of the antibacterial effect of silver ions on Escherichia coli and Staphylococcus aureus." J Biomed Mater Res, 2000; 52:662-668.

68) Bragg PD and Rainnie DJ. "The effect of silver ions on the respiratory chain of Escherichia coli." Journal of Microbiology, 1974; 20:883-889.

69) Chaw KC, Manimaran M, et al. "Role of silver ions in destabilization of intermolecular adhesion forces measured by atomic force microscopy in Staphylo-

coccus epidermidis biofilms." Antimicrobial Agents and Chemotherapy, 2005; 49:4853-4859.

70) Sondi I and Salopek-Sondi B. "Silver nanoparticles as antimicrobial agent: A case study on E. coli as a model for gram-negative bacteria." Journal of Colloid and Interface Science, 2004; 275:177-182.

71) DuHamel BG. "Electric metallic colloids and their therapeutic applications." Lancet, 1912; 40:89-90.

72) Morones JR, Elechiguerra JL, et al. "The bactericidal effect of silver nanoparticles." Nanotechnology, 2006; 16:2346-2353.

73) Yamanaka M, Hara K, et al. "Bactericidal actions of a silver ion solution on Escherichia coli, studied by energy-filtering transmission electron microscopy and proteomic analysis." Applied and Environmental Microbiology, 2005; 71:7589-7593.

74) Elechiguerra JL, Burt JL, et al. "Interaction of silver nanoparticles with HIV-1." Journal of Nanotechnology, 2005; 3:3-13.

75) Choi O and Hu Z. "Size dependent and reactive oxygen species related nanosilver toxicity to nitrifying bacteria." Environmental Science and Technology, 2008; 42:4583-4588.

76) Albrecht-Buehler G. "Rudimentary form of cellular 'vision.'" Proc Natl Acad Sci, 1992; 89:8288-8292.

77) Albrecht-Buehler G. "Cellular infrared detector appears to be contained in the centrosome." Cell Motility and Cytoskeleton, 1994; 27:262-271.

78) Albrecht-Buehler G. "Changes of cell behavior by near-infrared signals." Cell Motility and the Cytoskeleton, 1995; 32:299-304.

79) Litovitz TA, Mullins JM, et al. "Effect of coherence time of the applied magnetic field on ornithine decarboxylase activity." Biochem Biophys Res Comm, 1991; 178:862-865.

80) Litovitz TA, Krause D, et al. "Simultaneous applications of a spatially coherent noise field blocks the response of cell cultures to a 60 Hz electromagnetic field." In: Blank M Electricity and Magnesium in Biology and Medicine. San Francisco Press Inc, 1993.

81) El Sayed SO and Dyson M. "Comparison of the effect of multiwavelength light produced by a cluster of simiconductor diodes and of each individual diode on mast cell number and degranulation in intact and injured skin." Lasers in Surgery, 1990; 10:559.

82) Longo L, Evangelista S, et al. "Effect of diode laser silver arsenide-aluminum (GA-AL-AS) 904 NM on healing of experimental wounds." Laser Surgery Medicine, 1987; 7:444.

83) LAM TS, Abergel CA, et al. "Laser stimulation of collagen synthesis in human skin fibroblast cultures." Laser Life Science, 1986; 1:61.

84) Karu T, Andrelchuk T, et al. "Changes in oxidative metabolism of murine spleen following laser and superluminous diode (550- 950 nm) irradiation: Effects of cellular composition and radiation parameters." Laser in Surgery and Medicine, 1993; 13:453.

85) Young S, Bolton P, et al. "Macrophage responsiveness to light therapy." Laser in Surgery and Medicine, 1989; 9:497.

86) Feldherr C and Akin D. "The permeability of nuclear envelope in dividing and nondividing cell cultures." J Cell Biol, 1990; 111:1-8.

87) Feldherr C and Akin D. "Signal-mediated nuclear transport in proliferating and growth-arrested BABB/c 3T3 cells." J Cell Biol, 1991; 115:933-939.

88) Zhao Z, Wakita T, et al. "Inoculation of plasmids encoding Japanese encephalitis virus PrM-E proteins with colloidal gold elicits a protective immune response in BALB/c mice." Journal Virol, 2003; 77:4248-4260.

89) Simmons SR and Albrecht RM. "Probe size and bound label conformation in colloidal gold-ligand labels and goldimmunolables." Scan El Micr, 1989; 3:27-34.

90) Freund PL and Spiro M. "Colloidal catalyst: The effect of sol size and concentration." J Phys Chem, 1985; 89:1074-1077.

91) Skosey JL. "Gold compounds and D-penicillamine." In: Arthritis and Allied Conditions. McCarty DJ and Koopman WJ, editors. Lea & Febiger, Publishing, 1993; 603-614.

92) Shaya SY and Smith CW. "The effects of magnetic and radiofrequency field on the activity of lysozyme." Collective Phenomena, 1977; 2:215.

93) Ghadially FN, Oryschak AF, et al. "Ultrastructural changes produced in rheumatoid synovial membrane by chrysotherapy." Ann Rheum Dis, 1976; 35:67-72.

94) Salnikov V, Lukyánenko YO, et al. "Probing the outer mitochondrial membrane in cardiac mitochondria with nanoparticles." Biophysical Journal, 2007; 92:1058-1071.

95) Lewis C. "Die wirking von schwermetallen auf die bosartigen tiergeschwulste." Berl Klin Wochschr, 1913; 50:541-542.

96) Alekhina RP, Bukhman VM, et al. "Ratio between proliferating and quiescent spleen cell populations during development of Rauscher leukemia and after loading of mononuclear phagocytes with colloidal gold." Biull Eksp Biol Med, 1984; 97:790-793.

97) Mukherjee P. "Potential therapeutic application of gold nanoparticles in B-chronic lymphocytic leukemia (BCLL); Enhancing apoptosis." J Nanobiotechnology, 2007; 10.1186:1477-3155.

98) Bhattacharya R. "Gold nanoparticles inhibit VEGF165-induced proliferation of HUVEC cells." Nanolett, 2004; 4:2479-2481.

99) Mukherjee P, et al. "Antiangiogenic properties of gold nanoparticles." Clin Cancer Res, 2005; 11(9).

100) Bajaj S and Vohora SB. "Analgesic activity of gold preparations used in Ayurveda & Unani-Tibb." Indian J Med Res, 1998; 108:104-111.

101) Hillyer JF and Albrecht RM. "Gastrointestinal persorption and tissue distribution of differently sized colloidal gold nanoparticles." Journal of Pharmaceutical Sciences, 2001; 90:1927-1936.

102) Gottlieb NL. "Metabolism and distribution of gold compounds." J Rheumatol, 1979; 6:2-6.

103) Blocka KLN, Paulus HE, et al. "Clinical pharmacokinetics of oral and injectable gold compounds." Clinical Pharmacokinetics, 1986; 11:133-143.

104) Perrelli G and Piolatto G. "Tentative reference values for gold, silver, and platinum: Literature data analysis." The Science of the Total Environment, 1992; 120:93-96.

105) Campbell JM, Reglinski J, et al. "Action of sodium aurothiomalate on erythrocyte membrane." Annals of the Rheumatic Diseases, 1992; 51:969-971.

106) Tencer J, et al. "Size-selectivity of the glomerular barrier to high molecular weight proteins: Upper size limitations of shunt pathways." Kidney Int, 1998; 53:709-715.

107) Tay M, et al. "Charge selectivity in kidney ultrafiltration is associated with glomerular uptake of transport probes." Am J Physiol Renal Physiol, 1991; 260: F549-F554.

108) Rosenman KD, Moss A, et al. "Clinical implications of exposure to silver nitrate and silver oxide." Journal of Occupational Medicine, 1979; 21:430-435.

109) Cox AJ and Marich KW. "Gold in the dermis following gold therapy for rheumatoid arthritis." Arch Dermatol, 1973; 108:655-657.

**For further reading on the subject of alchemy:**

Atwood, A Suggestive Inquiry into the Hermetic Mastery, 1850

Hitchcock, Remarks on Alchemy and the Alchemists, Boston, 1857

Waite, Lives of the Alchemystical Philosophers, London, 1888

"   The Occult Sciences, London, 1891

Bacon, Mirror of Alchemy, 1597

S. le Doux, Dictionnaire Hermetique, 1695

Langlet de fresnoy, Histoire de la Philosophie Hermetique, 1792

"     "     Theatrum Chemicum, 1662 Valentine, Triumphal

Chariot of Antimony, 1656

Redgrove, Alchemy Ancient and Modern

Figuier, L'Alchimie et les Alchimistes, Paris, 1857

Made in United States
Troutdale, OR
06/18/2024